Research Tradition in Occupational Therapy

Process, Philosophy, and Status

Written by Charlotte Brasic Royeen
With a chapter by Gail H. Maguire
and a foreword by Elnora A. Gilfoyle

SLACK Incorporated, 6900 Grove Road, Thorofare, New Jersey 08086

Printed in the United States of America

Library of Congress Catalog Card Number: 87-043326

ISBN: 1-55642-035-8

Published by: SLACK Incorporated
               6900 Grove Rd.
               Thorofare, NJ 08086

Last digit is print number: 10 9 8 7 6 5 4 3 2 1

CONTENTS

Foreword

Acknowledgments

Author's Note

Overview

AUTHOR'S NOTE

I strongly believe in occupational therapy as a way to enhance the quality of life that all humans deserve. Moreover, I view research in occupational therapy as one way to help assure, through validation of practice and development of a body of knowledge unique to the field, that all in need have access to occupational therapy services. Therefore, it is my hope that this book will further foster interest in research on part of occupational therapists, and generate support for the tradition of research in occupational therapy.

Research is the "scholarly or scientific investigation" (American Heritage Dictionary, 1982, p. 1051). Tradition is the "pattern of thought or action" (American Heritage Dictionary, 1982, p. 1228). Hence, research tradition in occupational therapy is the manifestation of patterns and characteristics of scientific investigation, as well as thoughts or values underlying the research tradition. It is the tradition of research in occupational therapy that this book begins to address.

This book will not train someone to be a researcher. Rather, it is geared to familiarize the interested occupational therapist to the values, attitudes, and conceptualizations underlying research in general and occupational therapy research specifically. It is, in fact, an introduction to research in occupational therapy from a philosophical, global viewpoint by considering (a) research, (b) the relationship between research and clinical practice, (c) a humanistic foundation for research in occupational therapy, and (d) current and future trends and status of occupational therapy research. Furthermore, the book incorporates and reflects, as appropriate, current thought and controversy in related academic disciplines in regard to research.

Charlotte Brasic Royeen
Great Falls, Virginia, 1988

FOREWORD

Society's increasing complexity, the expanding web of social and health issues, and the multiplying of sub-specializations within health-related professions exacerbate the mandate for occupational therapy to develop its scientific base. A priority in occupational therapy today is to develop its academic base through conduct and utilization of research. Including research as a stated priority is not new; however, committing substantial resources for research endeavors is not only new but urgent. Occupational therapy can no longer justify its existence by stated personnel needs, or the inclusion of its services in laws, regulations, and accreditation standards. The profession must also establish itself as a science whose research undergrids the use of occupation in the promotion of health and life satisfaction. Thus, we must further develop the tradition of research in occupational therapy through the occupational therapy research consumer and the research therapist.

Christiansen (1986) delineated four requirements for facilitating the development of occupational therapy into a mature academic discipline:

1) Involving more people in the research endeavor,

2) Committing resources commensurate with the importance of the goal,

3) Raising our expectations with respect to research involvement and awareness, and

4) Reducing the ambiguity of our domain of knowledge (p. 324)."

Unfortunately, occupational therapy does not have many clinicians or faculty members whose training and major time commitments are in research. Recent estimates from survey data indicate that fewer than 2% of occupational therapy clinicians identify research as part of their responsibilities, with only .04% identifying research as their primary role. In a recent study, Parham (1985) reported that over 50% of occupational therapy faculty teaching at research universities had not published a single article in a refereed journal.

Inadequate personnel resources are accompanied by limited financial resources available for occupational therapy research. Although there is a strong commitment to research by both private and public sectors, grant-supported research in occupational therapy is miniscule. The American Occupational Therapy Association has spent less than 5% of its annual budget on research activities, which further exacerbates limited financial resources (Gilfoyle, 1986).

The profession's educational standards require entry-level programs to involve a "critique of studies related to occupational therapy" and "the application of research approaches to occupational therapy practice" (American Occupational Therapy Association, 1983, p. 3). Therefore, the entry level requirements promote development of the occupational therapy research consumer. These standards apply to students entering programs at the graduate and undergraduate levels. Unfortunately, occupational therapists can earn graduate degrees by acquiring the same minimal standards as those receiving baccalaureate degrees. As stated by Christiansen (1986), these standards pose a problem: "By permitting nonthesis options in our graduate curricula, we are communicating in a symbolic way that research does not hold a high priority, and we are depriving the field of the socialization experiences so vital to the young scientist-practitioner" (p. 336).

The need to increase our resources for research activities is critical. The requirements, cited by Christiansen (1986), deserve special attention with the development of strategies and action plans to achieve that goal. We need to further develop the tradition of research in occupational therapy. One strategy vital to increased resources is the development and publication of literature addressing research endeavors.

Considering that research is a critical but perhaps unpopular endeavor, I commend the author and publisher for their foresight in providing us with this valuable publication on the tradition of research in occupational therapy. This book will serve as an important contribution to occupational therapy, and perhaps, to other health-related disciplines interested in it as a prototype. The material in the text is a unique, refreshing approach that renders the process, philosophy, and status of research in occupational therapy comprehensible and viable for occupational therapy research consumers and research therapists alike. The author presents information that is useful to students, clinicians, and educators. Hopefully the text will serve as an impetus to excite others in becoming active participants in the research endeavor as either research consumers or research therapists.

This book can be viewed as a "pioneering publication," as the author has presented research and occupational therapy as a federation, rather than research in occupational therapy as an isolated subject matter.

Elnora M. Gilfoyle
President, American Occupational Therapy Association, 1986 - 1989

REFERENCES

American Occupational Therapy Association (1983). Essentials for an accredited program for the occupational therapist. Rockville, MD.

Christiansen, C. H. (1986). Research as reclamation. Occupational Therapy Journal of Research, 6, 323-327.

Gilfoyle, E. M. (1986). Professional directions: Management in action. American Journal of Occupational Therapy, 40, 593-597.

Parham, D. P. (1985). Academic reward structures and occupational therapy faculty. Part I: Characteristics of faculty. Occupational Therapy Journal of Research, 4, 83-100.

American Heritage Dictionary, 2nd Ed. (1982). Boston, MA: Houghton Mifflin Co.

ACKNOWLEDGMENTS

The author wishes to acknowledge A. Matin Royeen, Ph.D., for assistance in development of many of the concepts presented in Chapter Two.

Comments by Dr. Jim C. Fortune on his analysis of occupational therapy research design have been adapted by the author, and Dr. Fortune's influence is acknowledged.

Parts of Chapter Four are taken from "The Boxplot: A Test for Screening Research Data" (American Journal of Occupational Therapy), Vol. 40, No. 8, p. 569-571, 1986) by C. B. Royeen and adapted with permission.

This book was prepared by the author in her private capacity. No official support or endorsement by the U.S. Department of Education is intended or should be inferred.

OVERVIEW

Chapter One of *Research Tradition in Occupational Therapy: Process, Philosophy, and Status,* "Research and Occupational Therapy," discusses why research is important in occupational therapy and presents characteristics of quality research as a method of evaluating research in occupational therapy. Chapter One also presents a model of the process of research for a conceptual framework of the research tradition in occupational therapy as related to theory and theory development.

Chapter Two, "A Humanist's Approach to Research," is a philosophically oriented chapter on humanism as a foundation of occupational therapy and as a foundation of the research tradition in occupational therapy. An argument for how occupational therapy research can be judged as humanistically oriented is put forth. Also, consideration is given to humanistic research, not just as a product, but as part of the process in which the investigator engages.

Chapter Three, "Research Design as Clinical Practice," by Gail Hills Maguire, delineates the move from occupational therapy clinician to occupational therapy researcher in a step by step process that includes explaining the relationship of research design to clinical practice. This is a practically oriented chapter predicated upon the similarity of the problem-solving process between research and occupational therapy practice. This chapter can serve as groundwork for the tradition of the research consumer as well as the research therapist.

Chapter Four, "Current State of the Art in Occupational Therapy Research," provides an overview of the status and current tradition of occupational therapy research by analysis of statistical procedures employed. Suppositions are presented based upon analysis of occupational therapy research literature.

Chapter Five, "Future Trends in Occupational Therapy Research," projects where future directions and traditions may be in occupational therapy research, considering current status of the field as well as current status of related disciplines of academic thought.

ABOUT THE AUTHOR

Charlotte Brasic Royeen, Ph.D., O.T.R., is a Research Analyst with the Division of Innovation and Development, Office of Special Education Programs, U.S. Department of Education. She graduated summa cum laude with a B.S. degree in occupational therapy from Tufts University, with a M.S. degree in occupational therapy from Washington University School of Medicine, and a Ph.D. in educational research and evaluation from Virginia Polytechnic Institute and State University. She was supported for doctoral level study, in part, by a doctoral fellowship from the American Occupational Therapy Foundation.

Dr. Royeen's research interests have centered upon sensory integrative processing in children, the development of research methodologies for clinical investigation, and professional development/program evaluation in occupational therapy. Dr. Royeen serves on the editorial review board of several journals and is a faculty member of Sensory Integration International. Dr. Royeen was honored to become a Fellow of the American Occupational Therapy Association in 1988.

ABOUT THE CONTRIBUTOR

Gail Hills Maguire, Ph.D., O.T.R., is the Graduate Coordinator and Associate Professor in the Occupational Therapy Department, School of Allied Health Sciences, Florida International University. She graduated with a B.S. degree in Occupational Therapy from the University of New Hampshire, and received a M.S. degree in Education from Southern Connecticut State University. She earned her Ph.D. in Human Development from the University of Maryland as well as a doctoral level certificate in Gerontology from the University of Maryland Center on Aging.

Dr. Maguire is the editor of the book Care of the Elderly: The Health Team Approach (Little, Brown & Co.) and the October, 1988 issue of Topics in Gerontological Research on the Environment. She has authored articles and chapters on aging and serves on the editorial review board of several journals. Dr. Maguire regularly consults and offers workshops to professionals and community members on aging issues.

Chapter 1

The Research Process in Occupational Therapy

Charlotte Brasic Royeen

CHAPTER OVERVIEW

This first chapter of the book addresses basic issues such as the need and purpose of research in occupational therapy and the definitions as well as categorizations of research. Guidelines for what constitutes quality research in occupational therapy coupled with appropriate examples are presented. Subsequently, the overall purpose of the book is discussed. Selected readings for different areas of research in which the reader may have further interest are presented in the last section of the chapter.

KEY CONCEPTS

- Importance of research in occupational therapy
- Data base
- Discipline of knowledge
- Professional development
- Basic vs. applied research
- Clinical research
- Quality in research
- Research process vs. product
- Stages of the research process

NEED AND PURPOSE

Why are research and a research tradition important to the discipline of occupational therapy? Most occupational therapists consider themselves to be practitioners, and deem research to be an irrelevant, impractical, and unnecessary process not directly related to their primary concern of service delivery. Thus, many occupational therapists would answer that research is not important to a "real" occupational therapist, i.e., a practitioner who is rendering direct services on a regular basis.

However, it is for the occupational therapist who renders direct service on a regular basis that research is most important. Such individuals are professionally and personally committed to providing effective occupational therapy services in the most cost efficient manner and, therefore, need to be research consumers. Delivery of efficient and cost effective occupational therapy services should be predicated upon use and consumption of what Gillette refers to as a "data base" (1982). A data base is an empirically derived collection of knowledge about most aspects of a system, process, or, in this case, the practice of a profession.

Occupational therapy, though logically and intuitively on target, does not have an empirically derived data base demonstrating its appropriateness. Thus, we cannot demonstrate the effectiveness and efficiency of our practice to consumers, lawmakers, or academicians in the basic and social sciences. Gillette states:

> The established procedures of scientific investigation are the usual methods that follow when developing such a data base. Both qualitative and quantitative methods will be required if occupational therapy is to achieve its potential value in American society. (p. 499, Gillette, 1982).

Generation of a data base may also constitute generation of knowledge which is discipline specific. When a data base evolves from and relates to theory or theories, development of the data base does, in fact, contribute to the development of a "discipline." That is, disciplinary knowledge acquired from the process of generating a data base is that which makes such professions as medicine, anthropology, education, and psychology disciplines of science as well as professions. Development of a data base in occupational therapy will allow for concurrent development of the profession as a discipline of knowledge. Therefore, the end product of research in occupational therapy will be a data base about human engagement in activity.

Occupational therapy is not alone in this professional metamorphosis; nursing is in a similar situation. Like occupational therapy, nursing has been built upon knowledge from other disciplines in the basic and social sciences, and nursing is also in the process of developing a data base from original research within the profession (Wilson-Barnett, 1983). By observing the professional development of another field, and noting how our development mirrors it, the similarity of the process underlying the progression toward a data base and discipline of knowledge is apparent. Also, it is apparent that the progression is part of a developmental process inherent in the development of a profession into disciplinary status.

Development of a data base in occupational therapy would allow for the concurrent development of occupational therapy as a discipline of knowledge as alluded to by Yerxa and Sharrot (1986). Consequently, stating that occupational therapy research will allow for development of a data base on occupational engagement as well as disciplinary status for the profession is a valid answer to the question, "Why is research important?" However, a more compelling and humanistic rationale can be presented as an answer to inquiry regarding the importance of research in occupational therapy.

The need to know more and better ways to evaluate and intervene when infants, children, or adults experience occupational dysfunction is a drive as intense and basic as any in professional practice. Every occupational therapist has questions which evolve out of clinical practice. The following is a listing of example research issues/questions that have arisen from clinical practice.

Given two children with approximately equal degrees of tactile defensiveness, why can one child better mask or control behaviors related to tactile defensiveness when compared to the other child?

Which clients most need individual treatment sessions, and which would do well in group treatment sessions?

Why can certain severely dyspraxic children accomplish seemingly impossible tasks such as riding a bike or playing soccer?

Would encouraging upright or vertical postures prior to acquisition of basic prone and supine patterns reduce the development of spasticity in postcerebral vascular accident adults?

Would the development and refinement of adult level play skills in the person displaying a classic alcoholic personality reduce the recidivism rate?

How can occupational engagement of the elderly be enhanced from a macroperspective, i.e., communitywide, and can the effectiveness be documented?

Would a carefully designed prenatal program of sensory motor experiences benefit babies of highrisk mothers?

Dunn (1985) and Jantzen (1981) suggest that research is simply a way to find answers to such practice-driven questions.

DEFINITION AND CATEGORIZATION
OF RESEARCH

Given the purpose and need for research, we must define it. Simply stated, research is one or more activities based upon scientific procedures (Jantzen, 1981) employed to gather data and generate knowledge. Scientific procedures are guidelines or strategies which structure the process of research.

There are a variety of ways to categorize or "pigeon-hole" research. One of the most common and best understood categorizations is that of basic vs. applied research. Yerxa (1981) defines basic research as that which develops new knowledge, and applied research as that which has immediate benefits, meaning that it can immediately be applied for practical use. The distinction between basic and applied research can be blurred and somewhat artificial depending upon the actual nature of the research investigation. Examples of basic and applied research from the occupational therapy literature are presented in Tables 1-1 and 1-2.

Table 1-1.
Examples of Basic Research
in Occupational Therapy

Research Investigation	Topic of Investigation
Bowman and Katz (1984)	Studied hand strength and prone extension patterns in normal children
Cermack, Ward and Ward (1986)	Studied the correlation between motor coordination and articulation disorders in children
Kielhofner, Baus, Bauer, Shoestock and Walker (1983)	Studied play behavior in hospitalized and non-hospitalized children
Royeen and Kannegieter (1984)	Studied textural perception in normal children

Table 1-2.
Examples of Applied Research
in Occupational Therapy

Research Investigation	Topic of Investigation
Fisher, Mixon and Herman (1988)	Studied the validity of a clinical diagnosis of vestibular dysfunction
Smith, Cunningham and Weinberg (1986)	Studied the ability of *Functional Capacities Scale* to predict when a client could return to work
Storey, Bates, McGhee and Dycus (1984)	Studied the effectiveness of a program designed to reduce self stimulation in a retarded female

Table 1-1 demonstrates that the primary intent of the examples related to basic research is acquisition of knowledge related to phenomena or behaviors. Though the finding(s) may have clinical application, that is not the primary intent of the investigations. Compare this to examples of applied research presented in Table 1-2. Each of these examples has, as a primary intent, acquisition of knowledge which is directly clinically applicable. However, common to both basic and applied research is (a) presence of research issues or question to guide the research, (b) contribution to theory development or refinement, and (c) the need for each in occupational therapy (Yerxa, 1981).

A different way to consider research is a categorization of some subset of investigations as clinical research. Clinical research may be considered as:

>...clinical action executed with primary intent of creating generalizable knowledge; that is, the planned and systematic study of any clinical technique in an effort to support or discover its therapeutic effectiveness (National Commission of the Protection of Human Subjects of Biological and Behavioral Research cited on p. 407, Sharrot, 1985).

Clinical research may be considered to be a specialized form of applied research, having some unique characteristics (Royeen, 1986). First, clinical research employs subjects identified as deviating from "normal" in some systematic way, even if a control or comparison group is composed of normal subjects. Second, clinical research centers on questions which, when answered, will influence either evaluation or treatment of individuals characterized by a particular deviation from normal. In other words, clinical research centers on questions or phenomena related to theory which is directly related to or influences practice. Finally, clinical research is usually based upon relatively small samples since acquisition of subjects with identified and specified deviations from the norm is often difficult.

Clinical research in occupational therapy may be considered different from occupational therapy research. Whereas clinical research in occupational therapy concerns the practice of the profession or theories underlying practice, occupational therapy research concerns research into the profession itself. Examples of occupational therapy research studies follow in Table 1-3.

Table 1-3. Examples of Occupational Therapy Research	
Research Investigation	**Topic of Investigation**
Coleman (1984)	Studied development of the profession of occupational therapy in terms of a conflict between populist and elitist viewpoints
Parker and Chan (1986)	Studied perception of occupational and physical therapist regarding the degree of prestige associated with the professions
Royeen (1984a)	Studied the profile of therapists desiring certification in the sensory integrative testing

Table 1-3 suggests that a range of topics exist regarding researchable issues within the profession of occupational therapy. Just as both basic and applied research is needed in occupational therapy, so too, clinical research in occupational therapy and occupational therapy research are needed for development of the discipline and profession of occupational therapy.

QUALITY IN RESEARCH

Given the answers to why research is important and what constitutes research, another issue arises, pertaining to quality in research. Quality in research is extremely difficult to define since "...every study, no matter how sophisticated or well done, has some flaws or limitations" (p. 32, Polit & Heingler, 1985). Nothing in life is perfect and that most definitely includes research! Given the presence of the inevitable flaws or limitations in any study, what constitutes quality research?

Quality research is related to the decisions regarding research design which the investigator makes before implementing the study (Polit & Heingler, 1985). However, it also relates to the judgment based decisions the investigator makes about other aspects of the research during the study. For, just as quality treatment in occupational therapy relates to judgment decisions such as appropriate intervention strategies and monitoring of outcomes, the research investigator has to make judgment decisions regarding a variety of components of the investigation. It is the appropriateness of the research investigator's decisions that determines the quality of the research.

Still, however, the question remains: What constitutes quality research? Table 1-4 is a listing of the nine "components of quality research" to consider when evaluating the quality of any given research or research proposal. Each of these components will be discussed in turn.

Table 1-4.
Components of Quality Research

Number	Component
1.	Critical Issue
2.	Comphrehensive
3.	Competent
4.	Creative
5.	Cost Effective
6.	Context
7.	Common Sense
8.	Critical Flaw
9.	Communication

When evaluating clinical research in occupational therapy, one should consider whether the research addresses a critical issue: Is the research question or issue of importance, or is it investigating something not of particular significance to the field? The problem here is that significance, like beauty, is in the eye of the beholder. One has to assume a rather broad viewpoint and extend beyond discrete areas of interest to judge if, in considering the profession of occupational therapy as a whole, particular research attends to a critical issue. That is, does it attend to some aspect pertinent to the field even if it is not one's own specialty area or special interest?

Kirchman (1986) reported on an investigation into measurement of quality of life as enhanced by occupational therapy services. Her research most certainly addresses a key and critical issue confronting occupational therapy:

What is it that our services do? She has begun preliminary investigation into documentation of how occupational therapy services enhance quality of life given "...effects of losses" and "...deficits" (p. 21, Kirchman, 1986). Therefore, her research exemplifies orienting to a critical issue in occupational therapy research.

A second factor to consider when evaluating quality in research is whether the review, synthesis, and analysis of the literature pertaining to the issues or problems to be investigated is comprehensive. Has the investigator demonstrated a thorough and thoughtful understanding of the literature pertaining to the field of inquiry, in spite of space limitations that a journal publication may have in reviewing the literature? Are there omissions or misinterpretations of key articles or research directly relevant to the investigator's study?

An example of a comprehensive literature review in occupational therapy research is an investigation by Mathiowetz, Rogers, DoweKeval, Donahoe, and Rennells (1986). In their investigation of norms for the Purdue Pegboard Test, they present an appropriately detailed yet limited review of the literature pertaining to their investigation. The argument presented in the literature review is developed from broad concepts to very specific ones and is logically constructed. It is clear how the literature presented relates to their investigation and frames the research endeavor presented.

A third consideration is that of competence. Has the investigator demonstrated competence in all major areas of the research process? One might evaluate competence by posing the following questions:

Are the problems and issues leading to the investigation clearly identified and explained? Are the research questions and hypotheses (or equivalent tools in cases of qualitative research) clear and appropriate? Is the research plan or design appropriate and methodologically sound? Are the conclusions warranted and related to the research issue or question? Is the investigation competently related to some theory or set of theories?

An example of a competently executed research investigation is one by Oakly, Kielhofner, Barris, and Reichler (1986). In an investigation clearly related to the theory of occupational behavior, they present the development of an instrument designed to measure factors, in this case roles, pertinent to occupational behavior theory. The steps of the research are clearly presented. The research methodology employed is appropriate and well executed. Thus, one can answer "yes" to the questions posed related to the competency of the research.

A fourth consideration of quality in research is that of creativity. This is not a euphemism for making changes in data to guarantee significant findings or making interpretations not supported by or beyond the scope of the data. Rather, it refers to employing a unique perspective. For example, it is often difficult to investigate a certain problem because of methodological limitations. Does the research approach creatively solve that problem?

Sometimes, research results can be looked at in a new way which allows for significant theory development or modification. Thus, one might consider the following: Does the investigator offer insightful and creative interpretations?

An investigation by CooperFraps and Yerxa (1984) serves to illustrate an example of creative research. In this case, a creative interpretation was put forth and logically justified. They investigated social and sexual competence of burned, disfigured adults and found surprisingly high levels of social competence in certain victims. As an explanation of their unanticipated findings, they posed a creative explanation based upon the psychological mechanism of denial. That is, they suggested - and supported by selected literature - that denial may allow some severely disfigured burn victims to function at high levels of social competence. This is a novel way to explain their unanticipated findings and demonstrates that they interpreted research results in an insightful manner.

Cost effectiveness of the investigation is a fifth consideration of quality in research. Large samples, multiple groups, state of the art equipment, and release time to conduct investigations all cost money. Further, many, if not most, occupational therapy researchers are minimally funded, if at all. Thus, traditionally accepted research designs and procedures may be beyond the budget of most occupational therapy investigators. Consequently, it may not be reasonable to judge nonfunded occupational therapy research by standards of research appropriate for funded investigations. Therefore, a standard for evaluation of quality research might consider the financial resources available to the investigator and, given the degree of financial support, has the most been made of them and have valid results obtained?

Paired investigations by Gisel, Lange, and Niman (1984a, 1984b) serve to illustrate cost efficient research. Using the same control population of children and children with Down's syndrome, they investigated two distinct - yet related - areas of research; tongue movements and chewing cycles. This was cost effective since they did not have to obtain two separate samples. Yet, two preliminary sets of data were obtained on these distinct functions by employing the same sample twice.

A sixth characteristic to consider is context. Quality research takes results of the investigation and interprets them in the context of the numerous factors related to the phenomenon under study. For, just as no treatment situation occurs independently from the clinical setting, time of year, or family situation, research investigations do not occur in isolation. It is important that the context of the research be identified and considered, particularly when interpreting results of the study. As yet, no investigation exemplifies this type of analysis.

A seventh consideration of quality research concerns the often elusive commodity of common sense. Using a common sense approach, can one "map out" or logically delineate how the research issue, question, and design are all related? For example, does the reader obtain a common sense understanding of how the data obtained in the investigation is appropriate in order to answer the research question, or is the research issue, question, and data obtained seemingly unrelated? Sometimes, it is only after an investigation has been conducted that an investigator discovers that the data cannot answer the question posed, i.e., the wrong data was collected.

An investigation by Warren (1984) illustrates a common sense approach to research. She compared the apparent influence of the asymmetric tonic neck reflex in adults diagnosed as hemiplegic and a control group. By reviewing her publication, it is easy to see how her research question, issue, and design are related and to understand how the data collected (EMG recordings of muscle activity during varying postural conditions) yield meaningful information about her research questions. Thus, one has an easily obtained common sense understanding of her investigation.

The absence of a critical flaw is the eighth component of quality research. As previously stated in this chapter, all research has problems: No research investigation is perfect. However, imperfections or limitations in a study should not constitute a critical flaw that is, in fact, fatal to the validity of the investigation.

What are critical flaws? They are something, anything, that renders a study invalid or suspect. Examples of critical flaws are:

- No measure of instrument stability (test-retest reliability) when the instrument was specifically developed for the investigation, and it is used to measure change.
- No measure of inter-rater reliability when a nonstandardized instrument is employed in an investigation.
- Use of a standardized instrument with subjects differing significantly from the standardization sample.
- A poorly conceptualized and executed research plan for which research findings are justified under the guise of phenomenological or qualitative research.
- Use of a purposive sample in an investigation with corresponding claims of statistical generalizability vs. generalizability to theory.
- Over-interpretation of the research results above and beyond what can be prudently concluded.
- Execution of too many statistical tests with a given data set such that the error rate is unacceptably high.
- Execution of statistical tests inappropriate for the sample size.
- Faulty or inappropriate assumptions underlying conduct of the investigation.

This list is by no means exhaustive because fatal flaws can occur for any number of reasons. One way of preventing fatal flaws is peer review at all stages of research (Dunn, 1985). Submitting one's work to peer review or obtaining collegial feedback does not guarantee that fatal flaws will not occur. However, it does assure that work has been reviewed by a more objective person and allows for insight into possible problems before they are irrevocable.

As stated previously, almost all research has flaws or imperfections. Nevertheless, flawed research may still be valid and justified in terms of conclusions drawn from the research. Examples of flawed, but basically sound research, follow in Table 1-5. (The author has chosen to use her own work rather than use colleagues' work as examples of flawed research.)

Table 1-5. Examples of Imperfect Research In Which Findings are Basically Sound		
Research	**Purpose**	**Imperfection**
Royeen (1984b)	Identify frequency of atypical vestibular functioning in behaviorally disordered children.	Principle investigator served as evaluator of the subjects. Examiner bias was introduced.
Royeen (1985)	Modify existing instrument development methodology for use with children.	Pilot testing of items for language comprehension was executing with children from a private school whereas the scale was normed with public school children. Item validity was jeopardized.
Royeen (1987)	Gather preliminary data on a questionnaire for tactile defensiveness in preschoolers	A smaller number of teachers rated a large number of subjects with resulting artificial increase in internal consistancy of the scale.

Imperfections in research, like fatal flaws, are varied and common. There is a difficulty in discriminating between research with fatal flaws and those with imperfections because it is essentially a judgment call as to when one (research with imperfections) becomes the other (fatally flawed and invalid). It is a matter decided upon by the research investigator and, most importantly, by the reader and consumer of research.

A ninth and final characteristic of quality research has less to do with the research itself than with communication about the investigation. Is the investigation communicated in a clear and concise manner, or is it made unnecessarily complex, cumbersome, convoluted, and confusing? Quality research is none of these.

An article by Ayres and Mailloux (1983) serves to illustrate a clearly presented published research. They presented findings and a logical argument for the possibility that puberty may exacerbate the condition of autism. Their argument is clear and easy to understand, when it could have been a jargon filled, complicated paper. Thus, their research was clearly communicated.

So far, this chapter has identified the need for and purpose of research in occupational therapy, provided definitions and categorizations of research, and provided guidelines for consideration of what constitutes quality research. The purpose of this book on research in occupational therapy will now be addressed.

PURPOSE OF THE BOOK

In part, this book constitutes analyses of occupational therapy research regarding current and future state of the art as well as identifies the components of the process of occupational therapy research. Moreover, it is an analysis of current and future research traditions in occupational therapy, and an analysis of the process and philosophy of the research tradition in occupational therapy. This book will not train an individual to be a skilled researcher. There are numerous books already available in a variety of research areas, and some of these are recommended at the end of this chapter. Training in research may be best accomplished if preceded by "enculturation" in research, and not all occupational therapists are meant to train in research. However, all occupational therapists can become "encultured" in the attitudes, values, and processes of research which is fundamental for the occupational therapist who is to become a consumer of research.

To clarify, Yerxa and Sharrot (1986) define training in terms of its Latin origin "...trahere" which means to pull (p. 155, Yerxa & Sharrot, 1986). It is not the purpose of this book to "pull" individuals along into research competency. Rather, it is the purpose of this book to educate individuals in the field of research as specifically applied to occupational therapy by introducing them to (a) the concepts of research, (b) the process of research, and (c) a proposed philosophy of research in occupational therapy.

Yerxa and Sharrot define "...educate" from the Latin "...ducere," to lead (p. 155, Yerxa & Sharrot, 1986). Thus, this book should serve to lead interested occupational therapists into "...understanding and reflection" and "...ability to think independently" regarding research (p. 155, Yerxa & Sharrot, 1986). After reading this book, one should understand the essential nature of research as a problem solving/judgement/decision making process, that is not dissimilar to the process of clinical decision making. Moreover, one should have an understanding of research as a process - not just a product. In her book *Models of Practice in Occupational Therapy*, Reed (1985) discusses the need to emphasize the practice of occupational therapy as orientation to the process of occupation or activity in addition to the outcome of the process, i.e., the product of occupation or activity. Similarly, engagement in research commits one to the process of research as well as to a product from the research.

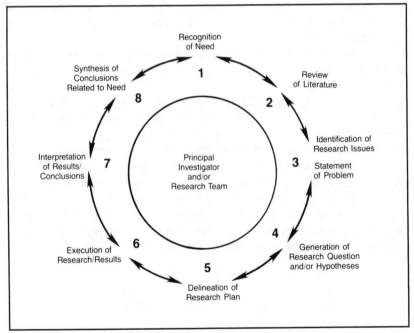

Figure 1-1. Overview of the stages of the Research Process.

15

Figure 1-1 is an introduction to research and presents the research process as a circular paradigm.

Figure 1-1 presents the research process as eight sequential stages from recognition of the need for research into a particular area to a synthesis of the conclusions from the research related back to the original need. This paradigmatic representation of research is simplistic and has been executed for purposes of clarifying the process. However, research as actually executed is not so discrete. The stages of research are not mutually exclusive. Like human growth and development, the stages of research are directional but may overlap. Indeed, one may at times even "regress" to an earlier stage, represented by the bidirectionality of the arrows in Figure 1-1. The center of the circle in Figure 1-1 is filled with the principal investigator or research team which reflects that research can be conducted by individuals or groups with a principal investigator overseeing the research.

Each of the eight stages of the process of research will be defined in sequence.

Stage 1. Recognition of a need to investigate some phenomenon in clinical practice, need to develop/refine instrumentation, need to study aspects of theory or the profession itself.

Stage 2. Review of the literature encompassing all published material directly and indirectly pertinent to the research need.

Stage 3. Identification of the research issues considering the need for the research in context of the literature review. Statement of the problem by summarizing research issues and focusing upon the problem area.

Stage 4. Generation of research questions and/or hypotheses based upon the statement of the problem.

Stage 5. Delineation of the research plan providing specifications for directing, interpreting, and coordinating the research. A schematic overview of content to be presented in the research plan is presented in Table 1-6.

Table 1-6.
The Research Plan

The research plan should include, but is not necessarily limited to statements on the following:

- Purpose and need of the study;
- Theoretical/conceptual basis underlying the investigation;
- Directional hypotheses where knowledge or experience permits;
- Description of research design including sampling plan which specifies units of analyses and sample definition/selection;
- Specification of dependent and independent variables;
- Plans for data analysis and conceptual rules for interpretation consistant with research issues and research questions being addressed;
- Measurement tools;
- Timeline of the study;
- Feasibility analysis of the investigation providing supporting evidence from the literature as to viability of design, measurement tools, etc., and as required a plan for pilot studies to establish feasibility of the study.

Stage 6. Execution of the research and results that consists of conducting the study, analyzing and verifying the data, and formating the results.

Stage 7. Interpretation of results/conclusions drawing upon disciplinary knowledge, theory, literature and creativity.

Stage 8. Synthesis of conclusions related to need incorporating the application of the interpretation to the original need driving the investigation.

The fact that research is a process and not just a product cannot be overemphasized. Research is a process whose end result can be tangible products such as manuscripts, theses, instruments or devices. Research products may also be "intangible" such as research results which change attitudes, alter or modify theories, or refine treatment procedures. Such intangible products may take years to manifest themselves.

In the subsequent and last section of this chapter, selected references in research are presented. This listing is not meant to be all encompassing, but it is meant to present references which are deemed to be especially useful and pertinent for research in occupational therapy. The reader is also referred to the reference section of each chapter for additional resources.

ITEMS FOR STUDY AND DISCUSSION

- Why is research in occupational therapy important?
- What is the relationship between a data base and a discipline?
- What is research?
- Differentiate basic and applied research.
- Define clinical research.
- Identify and define nine components of quality in research.
- Identify and discuss the stages of the research process.
- What are the "products" of research?

SELECTED READINGS

Computerized Procedures

Lefowitz, J. M. (1985). Introduction to statistical computer packages. Boston: Duxbury Press.

SAS User's Guide: Statistics. (1982). Carey, NC: SAS Institute.

SPSSx User's Guide. (1983). New York: McGraw Hill.

Evaluation Research

Kennedy, M. M. (1984). The problem of defining the problem. Evaluation Review, 8, 713-725.

LeCompte, M. D., and Goetz, J. P. (1982). Ethnographic data collection in evaluation research. Educational Evaluation and Policy Analysis, 4(3), 387-400.

Parente, R., and Anderson-Parente, J. (1986). Alternative research strategies for occupational therapy, part two: Ideographic and quality assurance research. American Journal of Occupational Therapy, 40(6), 428-431.

Royeen, C. B. (1986). Evaluation of school based occupational therapy programs: Need, strategy and dissemination. American Journal of Occupational Therapy, 40(12), 811-813.

Williamson, J. W., Ostrow, P., and Braswell, H. R. (1982). Health accounting for quality assurance. Rockville, MD: American Occupational Therapy Association.

Research Design

Benson, J., and Clark, F. (1982). A guide for instrument development and validation. American Journal of Occupational Therapy, 36(12), 789-800.

Ethridge, D. A., & McSweeney, M. (1971). Research in occupational therapy. Dubuque, IA: Kendall/Hunt.

Issac, S. A., and Michael, W. B. (1984). Handbook in research and evaluation. San Diego, CA: Edits.

Kerlinger, F. N. (1973). Foundations of behavioral research. New York: Holt, Rheinhart and Winston.

Ottenbacher, K. J., Barris, R., and Van Deusen, J. (1986). Some issues related to research utilization in occupational therapy. American Journal of Occupational Therapy, 40(2): 111-116.

Ottenbacher, K. J., and Bonder, B. (1986). Scientific inquiry: Design and analysis issues in occupational therapy. Rockville, MD: American Occupational Therapy Foundation.

Parente, R., and Anderson-Parente, J. (1986). Alternative research strategies for occupational therapy, part 1: Experimental and individual differences research. American Journal of Occupational Therapy, 40(5), 365-367.

Reed, K. L. (1984). Understanding theory: The first step in learning about research. American Journal of Occupational Therapy, 38(10), 677-682.

ShortDegraff, M., and Ottenbacher, K. (1986). Collaborative research in developmental therapy: A model with studies of learning disabled children. New York: Hawthorne Press.

Wilson, H. S. (1985). Research in nursing. Menlo Park, CA: Addison Wesley Publishing Co.

Qualitative Methods

Bogdan, R. C., and Biklen, S. K. (1982). Qualitative research for education: An introduction to theories and methods. Boston, MA: Allyn and Bacon, Inc.

Field, P.A., & Morse, J.M. (1985). Nursing research: The application of qualitative approaches. Rockville, MD: Aspen Publishing Co.

Glazer, B. G., and Strauss, A. L. (1967). The discovery of grounded theory: Strategies for qualitative research. New York: Aldine Publishing Co.

Goetz, J. P., and LeCompte, M. D. (1981). Ethonographic research and the problem of data reduction. Anthropology and Education Quarterly, Vol XII, No. 1, 51-70.

LeCompte, M. D., and Goetz, J. P. (1982). Problems of reliability and validation in ethnographic research. Review of Educational Research, 52(1), 31-60.

Kielhofner, G. (1982a). Qualitative research: Part one - paradigmatic grounds and issues of reliability and validity. Occupational Therapy Journal of Research, 2(1), 67-79.

Kielhofner, G. (1982b). Qualitative research: Part two - Methodological approaches and relevance to occupational therapy. Occupational Therapy Journal of Research, 2, 150-164.

Maanen, J. V. (1983). Qualitative methodology. Beverly Hills: Sage Publishing Co.

Merrill, S. C. (1985). Qualitative methods in occupational therapy research: An application. Occupational Therapy Journal of Research, 5(4), 209-222.

Parese, R. R., Coyne, A. B., and Smith, M. J. (1985). Nursing research: Qualitative methods. Bowie, MD: Prentice Hall.

Schmidt, H. (1981). Qualitative research and occupational therapy. American Journal of Occupational Therapy, 35(2), 105-106.

Single Case Study

Kratochwill, T. R. (1978) (Ed.). Single subject research: Strategies for initiating change. New York: Academic Press.

Ottenbacher, K. (1986a). Evaluating clinical change: Strategies for occupational and physical therapists. Baltimore: Williams and Wilkins.

Ottenbacher, K. (1986b). An analysis of serial dependency in occupational therapy research. Occupational Therapy Journal of Research, 6(4), 211-226.

Ottenbacher, K. (1986c). Reliability and accuracy of visually analyzing graphed data from single subject designed. American Journal of Occupational Therapy, 40(7), 464-469.

Statistical References

Box, G. E. P., Hunter, W. G., and Hunter, J. S. (1978). Statistics for experimenters: An introduction to design, data analysis and model building. New York: John Wiley and Sons.

Brunning, J. L., and Kintz, B. L. (1968). Computational handbook of statistics. Glenville, FL: Scott Forseman and Company.

Hinkle, D. E., Weirsma, W., & Jurs, S. G. (1979). Applied statistics for the behavioral sciences. New York: Houghton Mifflin Co.

Koopman, L. H. (1981). An introduction to contemporary statistics. Boston, MA: Duxbury Press.

Kotz, S., and Johnston, N. L. (Eds.) (1982). Encyclopedia of statistics. New York: John Wiley and Sons.

Mann, W. C. (1986). The choice of an appropriate statistic: A nonmathematical approach. American Journal of Occupational Therapy, 40(10), 696-701.

Ott, L. (1984). An introduction to statistical methods and data analysis. Boston, MA: Duxbury Press.

Salsburg, D. S. (1985). The religion of statistics as practiced in medical journals. The American Statistician, 39(3), 220-223.

Steel, R. G. D., and Torrie, J. H. (1980). Principles and procedures of statistics. New York: McGraw Hill.

REFERENCES

Ayres, A. J., and Mailloux, Z. K. (1983). Possible pubertal effect on therapeutic gains in an autistic girl. American Journal of Occupational Therapy, 37(8), 535-540.

Bowman, O. J., and Katz, B. (1984). Hand strength and prone extension in rightdominant 6 to 9-year-olds. American Journal of Occupational Therapy, 38(6), 367-376.

Cermack, S. A., Ward, E. A., and Ward, L. M. (1986). The relationship between articulation disorders and motor coordination in children. American Journal of Occupational Therapy, 40(8), 546-550.

Coleman, W. (1984). A study of educational policy setting in occupational therapy: 1918-1981. University Microfilms International, Microfilm #8421435: Ann Arbor, MI.

CooperFraps, C., and Yerxa, E. J. (1984). Denial: Implications of a pilot study on activity level related to sexual competence in burned adults. American Journal of Occupational Therapy, 38(8), 529-534.

Dunn, W. (1985). Occupational therapy's challenge: Caregiving and research. American Journal of Occupational Therapy, 39(4), 259-264.

Fisher, A. G., Mixon, J., and Herman, R. (1986). The validity of the clinical diagnosis of vestibular dysfunction. Occupational Therapy Journal of Research, 6(1), 3-20.

Gillette, N. P. (1982). A data base for occupational therapy: Documentation through research. American Journal of Occupational Therapy, 36(8), 499-501.

Giesel, E. G., Lange, L. J., and Niman, C. (1984a). Tongue movements in 4- and 5-year-old Down's syndrome children during eating: A comparison with normal children. American Journal of Occupational Therapy, 38(10), 660-665.

Giesel, E. G., Lange, L. J., and Niman, C. (1984b). Chewing cycles in 4- and 5-year-old Down's syndrome children during eating: A comparison of eating efficiency with normals. American Journal of Occupational Therapy, 38 (10), 666-670.

Jantzen, A. C. (1981). Research: The practical approach for occupational therapy. Laurel, MD: RAMSCO.

Kielhofner, G., Barris, R., Bauer, D., Shoestock, B., and Walker, L. (1983). A comparison of play behavior in nonhospitalized and hospitalized children. American Journal of Occupational Therapy, 37(5), 305-312.

Kirchman, M. M. (1986). Measuring the quality of life. Occupational Therapy Journal of Research, 6(1), 21-32.

Mathiowetz, V., Rogers, S. L., DoweKeval, M., Donahoe, L., and Rennells, C. (1986). The Purdue Pegboard: Norms for 14- to 19-year-olds. American Journal of Occupational Therapy, 40(3), 174-179.

Oakly, F., Kielhofner, G., Barris, R., and Reichler, R. K. (1986). The role checklist: Development and empirical assessment of reliability. Occupational Therapy Journal of Research, 6(3), 157-170.

Parker, H. J., and Chan, F. (1986). Prestige of allied health professions: Perceptions of occupational and physical therapists. Occupational Therapy Journal of Research, 6(4), 247-250.

Polit, D. F., and Heingler, B. P. (1985). Essentials of nursing research. Philadelphia: J.B. Lippincott Co.

Reed, K. L. (1984). Models of practice in occupational therapy. Baltimore: Williams and Wilkins.

Royeen, C. B. (1984a). Initial profile of therapists seeking certification in sensory integrative testing. American Journal of Occupational Therapy, 38(1), 44-45.

Royeen, C. B. (1984b). Incidence of atypical responses to vestibular stimulation among behaviorally disordered children. Occupational Therapy Journal of Research, 4(3), 59-60.

Royeen, C. B. (1985). Adaptation of Likert scaling for use with children. Occupational Therapy Journal of Research, 5(1), 59-69.

Royeen, C. B. (1986). An exploration of parametric vs. nonparametric statistics in occupational therapy clinical research. Doctoral dissertation, Virginia Polytechnic Institute and State University, Blacksburg, VA. University Microfilms International, Ann Arbor, MI: No. 8620659.

Royeen, C. B. (1987). TIP: Touch inventory for preschoolers - a pilot study. Physical and Occupational Therapy in Pediatrics, 7(1), 29-40.

Royeen, C. B., and Kanniegieter, R. A. (1984). Fingertip textural perception in normal children. Occupational Therapy Journal of Research, 4(4), 261-270.

Sharrot, G. W. (1985). Ethics of clinical research. American Journal of Occupational Therapy, 39(6), 407-408.

Smith, S. L., Cunningham, S., and Weinberg, R. (1986). The predictive validity of the functional capacities evaluation. American Journal of Occupational Therapy, 40 (8), 564-567.

Storey, K., Bates, P., McGhee, N., and Dycus, S. (1984). Reducing the selfstimulatory behavior of a profoundly retarded female through sensory awareness training. American Journal of Occupational Therapy, 38(8), 510-517.

Warren, M. L. (1984). A comparative study on the presence of the asymmetric tonic neck reflex in the adult hemiplegic. American Journal of Occupational Therapy, 38 (8), 386-392.

Wilson-Barnett, J. (1983). Nursing research: Ten studies in patient care. New York: John Wiley and Sons.

Yerxa, E. J. (1981). Basic or applied? A "developmental assessment of occupational therapy research in 1981. American Journal of Occupational Therapy, 35(12), 820-821.

Yerxa, E. J., and Sharrot, G. (1986). Liberal arts: The foundation for occupational therapy education. American Journal of Occupational Therapy, 40(3), 153-159.

Chapter 2

A Humanist's
Approach to Research

Charlotte Brasic Royeen

CHAPTER OVERVIEW

This chapter is a philosophical chapter which may be best approached by a process of reading, processing, and reflection. In other words, this may be a difficult chapter to read and will require more than one reading. The chapter begins with an introduction about occupational therapy in relationship to its humanistic origins. Subsequently, an argument is presented for how disciplinary needs are the impetus for research/statistical development in general, and in occupational therapy specifically. Humanistic research in occupational therapy is presented as one response to the disciplinary need. Finally, humanistic research in occupational therapy is defined and provisional guidelines for its conduct are presented.

KEY CONCEPTS

- Humanistic principals subserving occupational therapy
- Practice needs related to methodological development
- Research development in occupational therapy
- Humanistic research
- The reflective process in humanistic research

It was March of 1917 and the United States, under the leadership of Woodrow Wilson, had just become involved in World War I. In Clifton Springs, New York an important development also took place: The Society for the Promotion of Occupational Therapy was created (American Occupational Therapy Association, 1987). A group of six dedicated professionals, representing various backgrounds (American Occupational Therapy Association, 1987), created a profession whose members have, since its inception, effected many with commitment, dedication, and sincerity. According to West (American Occupational Therapy Association, 1987), prior to the creation of occupational therapy, patients with chronic, psychological conditions were locked away and were denied any kind of treatment. Modern awareness of occupational therapy "...came from the lower economic and indigent patients in almshouses and sanitoria who were given tasks to accomplish and were found to recover more quickly and completely than their wealthier counterparts who were constantly idle" (p. 24, American Occupational Therapy Association, 1987).

The term "occupational therapy" was created by one of the aforementioned dedicated professionals, a prominent psychiatrist named William Rush Denton (Bing, 1986). Denton's strong belief in training the sick or the injured by means of "purposeful activity" served as a legitimate foundation for treatment of patients or clients. Although purposeful activity may mean different things to different people, it is clear that occupational therapy emphasizes "doing" rather than "being." The values and principles of occupational therapy underlie the objectives of self-sufficiency and independence, i.e., to help the patient or client achieve to his or her maximum capacity. Achieve as used here does not mean "achievement of accomplishments," but refers to the ability to enjoy life to the fullest by realization of potential for quality of life.

Both the philosophy and practice of occupational therapy as manifested by practitioners are based upon a set of humanistic principles that cherish the best qualities of humankind such as loving, caring, tenderness, and sympathy. In the humanistic context, occupational therapy is concerned about the enrichment of human life to its maximum capacity through experimentation and practice and based upon engagement in activity, i.e., the science of occupation. By using activity, the occupational therapist attempts to transform disability or delay into function, and thereby, allow for individual fulfillment, feelings of worthiness, and meaningfulness of life.

A humanistic orientation can serve as a foundation for research in occupational therapy. However, a review of the historical development of research is necessary in order to set the context for a humanistic orientation in occupational therapy research.

RESEARCH DEVELOPMENT IN GENERAL

In an article identifying the relationship between context or issues/areas generating the need for research, and the corresponding statistical methodology employed, Box (1984) introduced the concept that practice influences statistics. (As defined here, practice refers to that phenomenon under study to which a statistical procedure is applied; it does not refer to the engagement in the art of occupational therapy.) To illustrate, Box (1984) cites the work of Gosset in which he analyzed small data sets from "...the laboratory, field trials, and the experimental brewery of which he was placed in charge in 1905" (p. 2, Box, 1984). Thus, the practice need (analysis of small data sets) led to Gosset's development of the t-test (a statistical/ methodological development) (Box, 1984). It may be that a humanistic orientation in occupational therapy research is a practice need which may similarly influence statistical/ methodological development in the future.

One of the earliest statistical tests of hypothesis was probably designed by Arbuthnot as a way to prove "divine providence" (Singer, 1979). In the middle ages, Arbuthnot used the sign test to demonstrate that for the preceding 82 years the actual rate of male births compared to female births was so outside the probability of chance that it had to be the result of "divine providence" and not accidental fate (Noether, 1980). Yet again, a practice need (analysis of male vs. female births in order to evaluate chance) led to a statistical test (the sign test).

Other similar patterns of statistical/methodological development related to practical needs can be identified. To illustrate, the work of Pearson is cited. He developed a form of correlational analysis and the corresponding concept of standard deviation in order to study characteristics of heredity (Johnston and Pennypacker, 1980).

In fact, much of the present day research design and corresponding statistical analyses have their origins in the work of Fisher, who investigated the differential effects of rainfall and other factors which affect agricultural plots of land (Box, 1984). It is clear that disciplinary practice and needs originating therein generate responses. These responses are the development of corresponding statistical procedures and research designs.

RESEARCH DEVELOPMENT IN OCCUPATIONAL THERAPY

Occupational therapy may be considered a disciplinary practice generating a need for statistical procedures and research methods. In this field, unique practice needs are inherent which challenge us to develop, refine, revise, and synthesize existing statistical procedures and research methods to meet our unique practice needs and professional values which are humanistically based.

Reed states that research design can "...provide the methods to examine multiple dimensions" (p. 48, Reed, 1984). Our challenge is to examine the multiple dimensions of variables and phenomenon of interest to occupational therapy in a way that appropriately considers the context of the investigation and employs a humanistic approach to the research process. The blending of a humanistic approach as part of the research design in occupational therapy research may be one way to meet the unique needs generated by our disciplinary practice. Given this overview of general research development and research needs in occupational therapy, concepts related to humanism will be further reviewed in order to prepare for a discussion of humanistic research in occupational therapy.

HUMANISM DEFINED

"Humanist" and "humanistic approach" are confusing terms having different meanings for different people. Such differences are related to the value system under which a person operates. To illustrate, "humanist teachings" as used by religious fundamentalists in Tennessee refers to teachings devoid of references to feminism, pacifism, and other "anti-Christian" themes (p. 1, Vobejda, 1986). In a more academic mode, humanism refers to a viewpoint of people "...based on the belief that the human organism is capable of self-regulation and self-maintenance that permit the individual to exert control over the environment" (p. 129, Reed, 1985). Such a humanistic theoretical reference is opposite to the mechanistic view based on the "...belief that humans function like a machine that must be regulated and maintained by the environment" (p. 129, Reed, 1985).

Humanism and humanitarianism have slightly different meanings. Humanitarianism refers to a concern for the welfare and interest of mankind. Humanism refers to a focus on distinctly human interests, but this focus does not have to be humanitarian. The humanist approach has been influenced by a number of different philosophical and religious thought systems that consider man as a conscious agent with feelings, ideals, and intentions.

Humanists believe that human beings are born with an inner nature composed of needs, talents, and anatomical equipment which, if allowed growth and expression, will develop and continue to grow in productive and healthy ways. Within a humanistic orientation, self-actualization refers to the actualization of inherent potential of one's inner nature. A self-actualized person knows himself or herself, is aware of his or her potential and his or her expertise, and acts in a manner consistent with his or her feelings. Within the humanistic context, an occupational therapist assists clients by closing the gap between the ideal self (what potentially exists) and the actual self (what the person really is).

Humanistic research as used here will refer to humanism defined in the more academic mode. Humanistic values and belief systems are consistent with the very origins of occupational therapy theory and practice. In fact, Reed suggests that humanism is the model upon which the early practice of occupational therapy was based, but that it's influence decreased until being revived in the 1960's (Reed, 1984). As an illustration of occupational therapy's early emphasis on humanism, Yerxa and Sharrot state:

Thus our predecessors viewed illness and disability as constituting special problems of daily living, and the new profession was designed to develop and foster the innate capacities of the person through engagement in occupation. Patients were conceptualized not as different from other people, but as people who had human needs in common with others and also needed to overcome unique challenges. This perspective placed the patient in the mainstream of humanity and within the universal human condition rather than in a diagnostic category or class. It also led to occupational therapy's basic questions of human existence: How shall I survive in the world? How shall I develop competence? How shall I make a contribution? (p. 154, Yerxa and Sharrot, 1986).

The orientation of occupational therapy to development of the self and the individual is consistent with an assumption of humanism: The assumption that there is an innate drive in an organism to increase autonomy (Woolpert, 1980). Thus, tenents of occupational therapy to reduce incapacity (Reilly, 1962), to improve quality of life (Kirchman, 1986), and to make doing possible are consistent with the assumption underlying humanism.

If self-actualization is the core of humanistic philosophy (Rowan, 1983), then self-actualization by doing is the core of occupational therapy. If, within a humanistic orientation "to be" is the key phrase of self-actualization, then "to do" is the key phrase of self-empowerment facilitated by occupational therapy. That is, doing is the manifestation, externally, of the process of self-actualization through engagement in occupation. In a sense, the "medium" (occupation) is the "message" (to do) (McLuhan, 1967).

A humanistic orientation is often assumed to be contrary to the scientific approach (Smith, 1982). That is to say, research and humanism are not considered to be compatible. However, academic educational approaches that employ humanistic orientations are not subject to this value judgment and are still considered academic teaching or instruction. The humanistic teaching approach is assumed to have the same content and outcomes of other teaching references, but it is the process that is assumed to be different.

If, indeed, it is the process which is different in humanistic teaching, then the same principle can be applied to research. To illustrate, the humanistic teaching approach has sensitivity to student needs as its first priority (Ryback and Sanders, 1980). Similarly, the humanistic approach to research need not be contrary to scientific processes; it may have sensitivity to the subjects as well as the investigator(s) as a priority.

Woolpert states:

> In the humanistic paradigm, there is a relationship between the objectified knowledge of imprecision and the personal knowledge of immediate experience ... In the humanistic paradigm, each way of knowing has a valid place. (p. 69, Woolpert, 1980).

Thus, in humanistic research the "objectified knowledge" as obtained through the scientific process can and should co-exist with the orientation to and active acknowledgment of the personal experience of subjects and researcher. The later is a humanistic orientation to research which occupational therapy can adopt.

Within the realm of neuroscience research, an experience the author had serves to illustrate this concept. Two researchers, Researcher A and Researcher B, were using rhesus monkeys for investigation. In order to perform microscopic analysis of the monkey brains, the monkeys were to be sacrificed at the end of the investigations. During the conduct of the investigation, Researcher A made a point of not becoming emotionally attached to the monkey, and, therefore, did not name it, attend to it, or play with it in any way. (This divorcement was not part of the scientific protocol of the investigation.) In contrast, Researcher B not only named the monkey, but interacted with it within appropriate confines of the research protocol, played with it, and oriented to it, not just as a research subject, but as a fellow creature on earth.

It could be surmised that Researcher A did not employ a humanistic orientation to research. That is, Researcher A could neither accept nor deal with the needs of the research subject (the rhesus monkey) within the confines of the research investigation and chose to deal with subject interactions as acts necessitated by "scientific" procedures. Contrast this behavior with that of Researcher B who had come to terms with the need to sacrifice the animal at the end of the experiment, and having accepted the need to do so, attended to the subject as a humanist and correspondingly oriented to the needs of the research subject during conduct of the study. Researcher B could accept the inevitable pain that would result from sacrificing the animal after developing an emotional attachment to it. Researcher A could not and chose to avoid it by denying the emotional needs of the animal. It is clear that in this instance the humanistically oriented Researcher B actively engaged in the self-awareness process germane to humanism and, therefore, allowed actions oriented to the needs of the subject rather than actions based upon self-interest.

Such a humanistic viewpoint of research, as exemplified by Researcher B, is broader and less rigid than what many individuals propose. Traditionally, humanistic research is considered to be that research in which the research question itself addresses content related to humanism. Such an approach is defined by Polkinghorne (1982):

Research is humanistic that addresses questions raised by considering people as agents who can act in a purposeful and meaningful manner. The logic of experience, as well as the logic of structures, can be used to clarify and extend our understanding of people as self-directing structures (p. 47, Polkinghorne, 1982).

Thus, humanistic research is traditionally defined as such because of the content of the research investigation. As proposed herein, humanistic research in occupational therapy would be so due to attitudes, values, and personal knowledge/examination that the research investigator effect in addition to addressing the research investigation itself which, eventually, will lead to a body of knowledge regarding human occupation. Humanistic research in occupational therapy would then clearly define, not just the theoretical context of the investigation, but also address the emotional and subject-centered content of the study. It is a viewpoint which assumes that humanistic research is a process and not a product of investigation.

In order to execute such humanistic research, an additional component of the research process must be executed: The reflective process inherent in humanism. The reflective process in humanistic research would consist of integrating the experiential approach with traditional methods (Price and Barrell, 1980). The experiential approach would be a "...scrutinization and clarification of one's basic attitudes, feelings, and values" (p. 28, Breck, 1976). This is what Researcher B in the example had accomplished and resolved.

How shall we accomplish humanistic research as exemplified by the reflective process in occupational therapy? Breck (1976) states that training in evaluation of ones values, feelings, and attitudes should be a prerequisite for training in research, especially experimentally based research. As a preliminary step toward identifying processes and procedures recommended for educating occupational therapists in humanistically oriented research, Table 2-1 presents suggested questions to guide the reflective process underlying humanistic research in occupational therapy.

Table 2-1.
Questions Underlying the Reflective Process
in Humanistic Occupational Therapy Research

Question Related to the Content of Research

1. How are the research questions for this investigation related to developing a data based on occupational therapy, i.e., related to knowledge on the process of engagement in occupation?

2. Why are these research questions important in terms of developing a body of knowledge related to occupational therapy?

3. Why are you (the investigator) interested in this?

4 What about the proposed research do you value and why?

5. What is your attitude regarding this research and how is it manifested?

Questions Related to the
Experience of Conducting the Research

1. What are your feelings about this research and why?

2. Is your behavior consistent with your feelings? Why or why not?

2. Are you sensitive to the subjects in the investigation? Why or why not?
   3a. If yes, how do you manifest your sensitivity?
   3b. If no, how is your lack of sensitivity manifest?

4. Are you sensitive to your own need regarding the conduct of the investigation.

5. Assuming any variety of possible outcomes or findings of your proposed research, how would you feel about each?

By attending to the preliminary guidelines presented in Table 2-1, humanistic research by occupational therapists will not necessarily result in publications based upon the reflective process or in specifically identifying the humanistic nature of it. However, it may well result in refinement and rigor in the investigator's conceptualizations of research processes and move occupational therapy further in the direction of integrated research. As a discipline, occupational therapy may be unique in that it, as both a theoretical (occupation science) and practice (occupational therapy) discipline, uses and relies on both a dichotomy of mechanistic and organismic models. By integrating a humanistic approach into our research process, we may further merge dichotomies, an integration which no discipline has yet been able to achieve. These dicho-'tomies are simplistically presented in Table 2-2.

Table 2-2. Dichotomies Based Upon Mechanistic Organismic Models		
Model	Mechanistic	Organismic
Foundation	Basic Science	Social Science
Predominate Process	Left Cerebral Hemispher	Right Cerebral Hemisphere
Way of Knowing	Deduction	Pattern Recognition
Thought Process	Linear	Multi-faceted

By integrating these two dichotomies, we would be realigning our interpretive models which could set exemplary standards for others to follow.

Moreover, by doing so, we could gain a modicum of power - for knowledge is power. In this case, the knowledge of how to integrate the two dichotomies of mechanistic and organismic models, and the power would be the enhanced strength of research in the profession resulting from such integration.

What would be the result of such power, and how could such power be reconciled with a humanistic approach to research?

A statement by Woolpert may hold the answer:

Power is not innately corrupting. It may, instead, have an enobling effect on those who yield it (p. 76, Woolpert, 1980).

ITEMS FOR STUDY AND DISCUSSION

-   How have practice needs influenced statistical/ methodological development in research?
-   Define humanist, humanism, and humanitarianism.
-   How is humanistic research traditionally defined, and how is it defined by this author?
-   What is the reflective process in research?

REFERENCES

American Occupational Therapy Association. (1987). The American Occupational Therapy Association at 70. Occupational Therapy News, 1.

Bing, R. K. (1986). The subject is health: Not of facts but of values. American Journal of Occupational Therapy, 40(10), 667-671.

Box, G. E. P. (1984). The importance of practice in the development of statistics. Technometrics, 26(1), 1-8.

Breck, L. A. (1976). Psychological research and humanistic values. North Quincy, MA: Christopher Publishing House.

Johnston J. M., and Pennypacker H. S. (1980). Strategies and tactics of human behavioral research. New Jersey: Lawrence Erlbaum Associates.

Kirchman, M. M. (1986). Measuring quality of life. Occupational Therapy Journal of Research, 6(1), 21-32.

McLuhan, M. (1969). The medium is the message. New York: Bantam Books.

Noether, N. E. (1980). The role of nonparametrics in introductory statistics courses. American Statistician, 34(1), 22-23.

Polkinghorne, D. (1982). What makes research humanistic? Journal of Humanistic Psychology, 22(3), 47-54.

Price, D., and Barrel, J. (1980). An experiential approach with quantitative methods. Journal of Humanistic Psychology, 20(3), 75-95.

Reed, K. L. (1984). Models of practice in occupational therapy. Baltimore, Maryland: Williams and Wilkins.

Reed, K. L. (1985). Views of humanity. In Planning and implementing vocational readiness in occupational therapy, M. Kirkland and S. Robertson (Eds.), American Occupational Therapy Association, Rockville, Maryland.

Reilly, M. (1962). Occupational therapy can be one of the great ideas of 20th century medicine. American Journal of Occupational Therapy, 16, 1-9.

Rowan, J. (1983). The real self and mystical experiences. Journal of Humanistic Psychology, 23(2), 9-27.

Ryback, D., and Sanders, J. J. (1980). Humanistic versus traditional teaching styles and student satisfaction. Journal of Humanistic Psychology, 20(1), 87-90.

Singer, B. (1979). Distribution-free methods for nonparametric problems: A classified and selected bibliography. British Journal of Mathematical and Statistical Psychology, 32, 1-60.

Smith, M. B. (1982). Psychology and humanism. Journal of Humanistic Psychology, 22(2), 44-55.

Vobejda, B. (1986). Fundamentalists prevail on texts: Students exempt from readings. The Washington Post. Saturday, October 25, A1, A7.

Woolpert, S. (1980). Humanizing law enforcement: A new paradigm. Journal of Humanistic Psychology, 20(4), 67-79.

Yerxa, E. J., and Sharrot, G. (1986). Liberal arts: The foundation for occupational therapy education. American Journal of Occupational Therapy, 40(3), 153-159.

Chapter 3

Research Design
as Clinical Practice

Gail Hills Maguire

CHAPTER OVERVIEW

The previous two chapters have introduced occupational therapy research with an overview and a discussion of humanistic approaches to research. This chapter will propose that viewing research design as clinical practice can assist the occupational therapist to develop the "mind-set" or research tradition necessary to function as the research consumer and the research therapist.

KEY CONCEPTS

- Research integration in clinical practice
- Problem solving as a foundation for clinical practice as well as research
- The clinically based research project
- How to recognize research topics/issues
- Similarity between a research plan and a treatment plan
- The "mind-set" or tradition of research

Anyone reading this book has probably been introduced to the argument that clinical research is important
to the future of occupational therapy practice. This chapter is designed to discuss practical issues in occupation
therapy research: Issues of how to move from cognitive
acceptance (research consumer) to actual involvement in
the process of research (research therapist) as identified in
Chapter One will be discussed.

Articles in the *American Journal of Occupational
Therapy* reveal that research has been identified as a
major priority of the profession since the 1960's, when
promotion of research to expand and validate occupational
therapy practice was a dominant theme (Kielhofner and
Takata, 1980). In the early 1970's, a series of six articles
by Ethridge and McSweeney covering major areas of clinical research were published in the American Journal of
Occupational Therapy (Ethridge and McSweeney, 1970a,
1970b, 1971a, 1971b, 1971c, 1971d). In their initial article,
Ethridge and McSweeney (1970a) stated that "occupational
therapy is not a 'research' profession. Rather, it is a field
of endeavor dedicated to the treatment or remedying of
human problems, and, therefore, our major concern is, and
rightly should be, professional 'practice' " (p. 490). However, they went on to say that as therapists seek answers
about treatment effectiveness, they are on the threshold
between "practice" and "research" (Ethridge and
McSweeney, 1970a). Ten years later, Kielhofner and
Takata (1980) identified that as an applied field, occupational therapy is most in need of applied research. Such
research includes identification of human problems followed by evaluation of the effectiveness of therapy programs.

In 1976, the American Occupational Therapy Foundation, in collaboration with the American Occupational
Therapy Association, sponsored a research seminar "...to
give impetus and substance to a national commitment to
research in the profession" (p. 509, Yerxa and Gilfoyle,
1976). At that time identified barriers to research were
attitudinal, organizational, and material constraints. Seminar participants offered general recommendations as follows (Yerxa and Gilfoyle, 1976):
-    Students and faculty should be more actively involved
     in research;

-   Clinicians and faculty needed to interact more frequently to conduct studies;
-   Rewards for doing research needed to be improved;
-   Complete and accurate data recording by clinicians should provide the foundation for many research studies.

Since that time, the American Occupational Therapy Association and the American Occupational Therapy Foundation have continued to foster research through various programs, fellowships, grants, consultations, and projects such as the publication of the teaching guide, "Integrating Research into Occupational Therapy" (Mitcham, 1985). Although improvements have been made in each of these areas in the past ten years and the foundation for research tradition in occupational therapy has been provided, all of the recommendations made at the research seminar are still applicable today. The main issue remains:

How can research be integrated as a clinical practice issue of the profession rather than remain as an issue of a select segment of therapists, i.e., how can a tradition of research become an integral part of the discipline of occupational therapy?

Webster's Dictionary defines a researcher as one engaged in research or the "...diligent inquiry or examination in seeking facts or principles; laborious or continued search after truth; investigation" (p. 715, Thacher and McQueen, 1967). Consider this definition for a moment, forgetting about the label "researcher." The description could very well define a therapist implementing the occupational therapy process: From the time of referral to discharge, the occupational therapy process requires a diligent investigation and examination of the facts, and a constant laborious search for truth that is similar to the research process. "Research needs to be perceived as part of the daily practice of occupational therapists, not research in the sense of full-time investigation, but research as it provides data for clinical problem-solving and decision making" (p. 8, Mitcham, 1985).

The first - and most necessary - step in the clinical research process is not learning a new technique, but acquiring a new mind-set. It is a mind-set which recognizes that clinical research is a natural function of practice, utilizing many of the same practice skills. It is the possession of practice skills combined with specific operating procedures i.e., the research process, that allows the move from research consumer to research projects developer.

In order to clarify how an occupational therapist can function as a research projects developer, the next section will identify and discuss the problem-solving approach as a common denominator subserving clinical practice and the research process. The steps in the occupational and research processes for purposes of this chapter will be defined, and the two will be compared in relation to problem-solving. The purpose is to demonstrate that by using familiar clinical problem-solving skills as the common link between the two, the clinician can develop the mind-set that research is a personal reality and a natural extension of the clinical occupational therapy process. Once this has been achieved, the steps and practical suggestions to design a research project in a clinical setting will be presented.

THE OCCUPATIONAL THERAPY PROCESS

For purposes of comparison to the research process in this discussion, the occupational therapy process is defined as: (a) receiving a referral - a patient or client is identified for occupational therapy; (b) data collection - including interviews and reviewing records; (c) evaluation - both formal and informal measures, to establish a base line of performance against which future evaluation results can be compared; (d) goal setting - defining and prioritizing goals based upon the evaluation results; (e) treatment planning - sequenced according to short- and long-term goals; (f) treatment - implementing the plan and adjusting it as necessary; (g) reevaluation - assessing progress, or the lack of it, against the baseline established by the most recent evaluation; (h) reporting - progress; and (i) either terminating or continuing the treatment. See Table 3-1 for a comparison of the two processes in relation to the problem-solving approach.

Table 3-1.
Comparison of Problem Solving in Occupational
Therapy Process and Research Process

Problem Solving	Occupational Therapy Process	Research Process
Problem Identification	1. Referral	1. Recognition of Need
	2. Data Collection	2. Review of the Literature
	3. Evaluation	3. Identification of Issues
	4. Goal Setting	4. Generating Questions/Hypotheses
Solution Planning	5. Treatment Planning	5. Research Planning
Solution Implementation	6. Treatment Implementation	6. Execution of Research
Solution Evaluation	7. Re-evaluation	7. Interpretation of Results
	8. Reporting of Results	8. Synthesis/Conclusions
	9. Termination/Continuation	9. Termination/Continuation

THE RESEARCH PROCESS

The research process outlined in chapter one will be further described as follows: (a) recognition of a need and identifying a research topic; (b) review of the literature and data gathering, including pertinent unpublished materials such as clinical forms; (c) identification of the research issues to determine the problem in light of the literature review; (d) generation of research questions or hypotheses based upon the statement of the problem; (e) delineation of the research plan to include selection of the sample, instruments, procedures, and methods to analyze the data; (f) execution of the research and results by following a standard operating procedure; (g) interpretation of results/conclusions to determine whether the results supported the hypotheses significantly; and (h) synthesis of conclusions related to need drawing upon theory and the implications for the profession. Termination, continuation, or adaptation of the research plan is an additional step that is often assumed, but not labeled as part of the research process.

THE PROBLEM SOLVING APPROACH

The nine steps in both the occupational therapy and the research processes have been delineated to demonstrate how similar the steps are. The important issue is how to make what may seem like a major leap from clinical practice to beginning or regular researcher or research consumer. Mitcham (1985) has suggested that the problem-solving approach which should be common to all occupational therapy practice and occupational therapy curricula can be the link.

In describing a problem-solving approach four steps are usually delineated: (a) identifying the problem, (b) planning the solution, (c) implementing the solution, and (d) evaluating the results. Mitcham states: "These four steps of problem-solving are evident in the process of conducting research and in the process of delivering occupational therapy services" (p. 12, Mitcham, 1985).

In stage one, "The Problem Identification Stage," screening and evaluation are required for both research and the occupational therapy process. Screening and evaluation for the occupational therapy process includes referral, data collection, and evaluation. In occupational therapy, long- and short-term goals and treatment objectives span the problem identification and the solution planning stages because they identify the behavior that needs improvement, but they also state the expected solution. Screening and evaluation for the the research process includes recognition of the need for research and topic identification, review of the literature, and defining issues. Identifying the questions or hypotheses in the research process also spans both the problem identification and solution planning stages in the same manner as goal setting does in the occupational therapy process.

Stage two, "The Solution Planning Stage of Problem-Solving" involves treatment planning for occupational therapy and delineation of a plan for research. Occupational therapy planning includes identification of goals and selection of treatment modalities. Delineation of a research plan involves selection of the methodology including appropriate tools, data collection, and analysis.

Stage three, "The Solution Evaluation Stage," constitutes the execution of the selected treatment in occupational therapy based on the treatment plan that includes implementation of the selected methodological procedures to collect the data following a standardized procedure leading to interpretation of results and conclusions.

Finally, Stage Four, "The Solution Evaluation Stage," is composed of the reevaluation, reporting of results, termination, continuation, and adjustment of treatment in the occupational therapy process. The research process includes analysis of the data, and interpretation of results and conclusions, termination, continuation, and adjustment of the research. Unlike clinical practice in which one reports the results and implications for just one patient, results in the research process are synthesized in relation to theory and clinical phenomena are generalized (Mitcham, 1985; Rogers, 1982).

DESIGNING A CLINICALLY BASED RESEARCH PROJECT

If from this comparison we can accept that the routine procedures followed in the occupational therapy process are very similar to the research process, then we can proceed to determine what steps are necessary to incorporate the design and implementation of a research project as part of clinical practice for those therapists who wish to move beyond the beginning research consumer to actually designing a research project (Mitcham, 1985, 1983).

RECOGNIZING THE NEED AND SELECTING A RESEARCH TOPIC

Earlier we discussed that the first step in accepting that all occupational therapists have a professional obligation to be researchers on some level is to develop a mind-set, to recognize that research is really a natural part of clinical practice. Underlying this recognition is an assumption that clinical practice is the primary foundation, and that research emanates from clinical practice. Subsequently, practice may or may not be modified based on the results of the research.

Thus, one of the first steps as a researcher is the identification of something worthwhile to investigate. Often, therapists will say they want to conduct research or write an article. The missing component in the statement is the "something" to research and report. Lack of a research idea may result from two possible, but not equally probable, explanations. First, there is nothing in the practice environment meriting investigation. Second, and more likely, is the inability to recognize problems within the practice environment which warrant investigation. This problem, identification, can be one of the most variable steps in length of completion time. Initially, however, it does not need to take more time than that which is normally scheduled in the clinic. To illustrate, if a specific issue to study does not immediately come to mind, keep a note pad in a pocket or in a convenient place and, as possible issues or problems arise, they can be easily recorded.

This technique is analogous to training dream recall by keeping a writing pad next to the bed and recording dreams upon awakening. This technique is one part of the mind-set to developing an awareness of research. It is similar to becoming a new parent or having tennis elbow. Once these issues become part of a personal reality, one suddenly notices, and even seeks out, others in similar situations. Furthermore, once one is oriented to research as a personal reality, identification of questions about everyday practice that may be answered by research comes more easily.

If one has very limited time in a department, one solution is to divide the responsibilities among several interested staff members and form a research team. For instance, one therapist could be responsible for designing the project, with input from the other participants through brainstorming meetings and reviewing the plans. Another therapist, or therapists if the department is large enough, could conduct the research, another could be responsible for coordinating meetings with a consultant to have the material analyzed, and one could write up the results with everyone editing the report. Weiss (1977) has suggested that cooperative research can increase the potential scope of the project, but factors such as variations in methods of data collection by different testers are potential problems that require carefully standardized methods.

REVIEW OF THE LITERATURE AND DATA COLLECTION

Once the topic has been identified, the next step is to do a preliminary search of the literature to discover what other people have written about the subject. Normally, researchers use the literature review to establish the significance of their research problem, and the potential contribution of their studies to the current state of knowledge in the field (Crocker, 1977). The literature review will continue as the research progresses to keep it current or as the need for additional information is identified. The literature review may lead to modification of the topic as more information is gained.

Delineation of the conceptual basis, including the theoretical framework, is necessary throughout the research process. Kielhofner and Takata (1980) suggest that when occupational therapy clinical programs are developed on the basis of a theoretical model, research designed to test the effectiveness of the program can also test and further expand the underlying theory. As early as possible in the literature search, authors can be contacted to request copies of instruments that may be helpful in the conduct of the proposed research. Permission to use their material must be obtained if it is copyrighted. Also, additional information from authors about how they conducted their study, including problems they may have encountered, can be requested. Authors are usually very happy to have someone duplicate a study or utilize their material as long as the work is properly referenced. In a request letter, it would be appropriate to ask the authors to spell out exactly how they want the credit to be written, including name and institution, and indicating that their material is being used with permission.

During this time, any unpublished material, such as pertinent clinical forms, can also be collected. Directly coping departmental forms or materials from books and journals without receiving permission or referencing the work is unethical and illegal according to the copyright laws. Even material that is not copyrighted but still obtained from another therapist or institution should be referenced. Also, be sure to specifically identify (name, title, date, institution) all material developed within a given project. That way future staff will know the author if they decide to revise the material or need additional information.

The literature review will require additional time in a work schedule. If your employer will allow library time, a couple of half days per week to get articles from the library will be needed. If a schedule is developed, articles can subsequently be read in small blocks of time. If it is difficult to get time away from the clinic, it is important to plan for and schedule time outside of work in order to get the initial review done. It is more efficient to try to get this step done within a concentrated time frame or momentum can be lost.

It can be very helpful to identify one or two colleagues with whom ideas can be discussed. This makes the whole process "real," and renders it in the frame of reference for your clinical practice. Often, just by talking through ideas and issues of research problems in this initial phase, the research plan is strengthened. Once sufficient information has been collected, and it is determined that a current overview of the topic is completed, it is time to progress to the next step.

IDENTIFICATION OF THE RESEARCH ISSUES

When the initial literature review is complete, one is better able to formulate the scope of the clinical problem for the study. A statement of the problem summarizing the research issues involved will be the basis for the formulation of the research questions and hypotheses.

DEFINING THE RESEARCH QUESTIONS OR HYPOTHESES

It is now time to determine exactly what research question(s) are to be answered.

Development of a researchable question requires three basic components which are also found in a treatment objective. These are, first, identify the terminal behavior or outcome, stating what will be accepted as evidence that the process has been completed. Second, define the activity or process through which the desired outcome is to be achieved. Third, specify the criteria of the research project (Ethridge and McSweeney, 1970a).

There are some practical factors to be considered as the research topic is crystallized. Determining what resources are available such as secretarial, computer, and public relations can be very important. For example, choosing a project that can be incorporated into the general clinical schedule may be the only practical choice. In addition, assessing available resources includes determining what funding is available. One may consider the possibility of other agencies or institutions wanting to share the

project and expenses. Or, if the administrator says research is important but the departmental workload is such
that he or she can not allow for any release from patient
treatment time, then negotiation of other resources which
may be available can begin. Choosing a research project
that the administrator identifies as important or that ultimately may be cost effective or benefit the institution can
be strategic!

Consistency and efficiency in implementation of the
research is very important. Evaluate the time schedule to
determine how management of data collection will be
implemented. For example, determine if the records and
information needed routinely are available. Don't decide on
a project that requires surveying family members unless it
is a routine part of the evaluation procedure. Considerable
free time can be spent tracking down family members and
still result in insufficient numbers. Further, keep the plans
as manageable as possible. Assuming that the research
question(s) have been developed, the next important part
of the research process is defining the research hypothesis.

The hypothesis is a statement about the relationship
between the dependent variable(s) or terminal behavior(s)
and the independent variables or treatments that carries
implications for testing the stated relationships, including
the expected outcome of the study. In other words, a hypothesis has to be testable. It is often helpful to construct a
couple of hypothetical cases of potential subjects to identify what variables must be considered before the hypothesis is written. The important factor at this stage is to list
all the variables that might impact on the study: Hypotheses will reflect the main relationships. It may require
some uninterrupted time to develop and refine the hypothesis. Keep ongoing notes as variables come to mind.

DELINEATION OF THE RESEARCH PLAN

If the previous steps have been followed, one has a
head start on designing the research for potential problems. Variables that are important to the study and the
hypotheses have already been identified. The next step,
careful planning of the research design, is crucial to a
successful project. Conine (1972) summarized Ethridge and
McSweeney (1971a) well in describing a research design:

50

Design is a blueprint that the researcher drafts to chart his course for testing the hypothesis. The researcher specifies the exact procedures to be used in drawing a sample from a clearly defined population, the method of assigning subjects to various groups, the instruments or tests to be used, and how the data will be analyzed in order to test the hypothesis (p. 82, Conine, 1972).

Definition of the population of subjects about whom the conclusions will be drawn is basic to early planning. Other literature covers methods to reduce the chance of bias in subject selection (often by assuring a statistically significant sample size), but a practical consideration is whether you will have a sufficient number of subjects to complete the project in a timely fashion.

Many experienced as well as new researchers have ended up taking much longer to complete their research, or have a smaller number of subjects to work with than they had expected, because they did not take into consideration the availability of appropriate subjects. Once the subjects have been defined and their selection specified, a complete definition of the independent and dependent variables is required. This can be followed by a description of the procedure that will be used to conduct the research and all tools and treatments which will be administered. The description must be specific enough so that someone else reading it would know how the procedures were designed. Writing each step of the research proposal will help clarify the thought process and identify missing information. It is also helpful to have someone unfamiliar with the project read the description of the research to see if it is complete and whether the procedures are clearly written. At this point, it is time to determine how the data will be analyzed once the research is completed. If assistance is needed with statistical procedures, it is helpful to team up with someone with such experience, such as a faculty member at a university. This is the time to delineate for the statistical expert exactly what is desired when the research is completed.

The measuring process or instrumentation should be characterized by validity (whether the instrument actually measures the identified variable) and reliability (consistency of measurement). Excellent descriptions of the various types of validity and reliability are covered in basic research or measurement texts and articles (Crocker, 1976; Ethridge and McSweeney, 1971b; Hasselkus and Safrit, 1976; Kerlinger, 1973).

In the occupational therapy treatment process there should be a treatment plan for every treatable deficit identified in the evaluation, or documentation which states why there is no plan. Similarly, in the research process, one should also account for all of the variables identified as significant to the project. A good plan for a research project should make the actual execution of the plan somewhat routine. For example, if one is going to administer an interview to every stroke patient who receives treatment in occupational therapy for a particular three-month period, then the interview form would routinely be included in all initial evaluations of stroke patients. Every subject would be interviewed utilizing a standard protocol, and the information obtained would be recorded in a uniform manner. One would also decide whether the subjects would be limited only to those who could speak or respond accurately, or if one would obtain information from a family member, which might require additional steps such as a preliminary screening test. Prior planning would insure that the forms were ready, and the therapists were trained to administer and record the interview in a uniform manner. No extra time would be necessary during the evaluation if most of the information was already obtained in various other formats. Piloting the actual procedure on a small sample of subjects who will not be used in the study is a good way to determine how the actual process works. The necessary adjustments should be made in the process before beginning the actual project.

A well designed research plan includes descriptions and samples of all of the materials and procedures necessary to begin execution of the plan. Finally, instituting a small pilot project enables the researcher to proceed through all of the steps to determine if the methodology is sound and manageable and to make any necessary adjustments.

EXECUTION OF RESEARCH AND RESULTS

In the course of the occupational therapy process, a treatment program is implemented based on the results of the evaluation process and the short- and long-term goals. In the same way, implementation of the research project may include administering the same types of treatments that are routinely done. The difference is that all of the relevant procedures must be administered and recorded in a uniform manner for all individuals who were previously identified as potential subjects. All information obtained for the study should be filed separately for the study or should be recorded in a manner so that the information pertinent to the study is readily retrievable.

INTERPRETATION OF RESULTS AND CONCLUSIONS

After the occupational therapy treatment program has proceeded for a period of time, the therapist will do a reevaluation to determine the results of the treatment program. Similarly, after the implementation of the research, the results will be analyzed to determine if the hypothesis was correct. This is usually done through a statistical analysis which may be as simple as computing the frequencies and means, or as complicated as multivariate analysis.

Analysis and interpretation of the data is influenced by the characteristics of the study that were set earlier. For example, one can not generalize beyond the population that is represented by the subjects. Likewise, results will be interpreted according to the relationships of the variables defined in the hypothesis. As was mentioned under the problem-solving process, the interpretation of results is the area of the research process that is the most dissimilar to the occupational therapy process. In the treatment process, the interpretation of results based on the reevaluation will only apply to the specific patient who was treated. Presentation of evidence supporting or invalidating the research hypotheses is incomplete unless the results in relation to the theoretical orientation and the relevant studies presented in the literature review are discussed. Identifying similarities and conflicting results will assist the reader to view the study in a broader perspective (Ethridge and McSweeney, 1971c).

SYNTHESIS OF CONCLUSIONS RELATED TO NEED

Documentation of research findings is more comprehensive than the treatment process where the therapist just reports the results after the reevaluation. Documentation of the findings include both the interpretation and synthesis steps. Madsen and Conte (1980) suggested that documentation does not have to be limited to research-oriented therapists; the development of empirical approaches to treatment promotes active participation of all practitioners. Just as in the treatment process, documentation is sometimes the most tedious part of research. All of the data that are pertinent to the hypotheses are reported in an objective manner; opinions and speculations regarding the results are reported as such. Statistical information is supplied to document the findings so that readers can make their own decisions about the results.

TERMINATION, CONTINUATION, OR ADJUSTMENT OF THE PROJECT

In the treatment process, a reevaluation offers the choice of whether to terminate, continue, or adjust the treatment. In the research process, often the project is of a known duration because of limits set initially by the researcher in the research plan or because of funding allocations; the project is terminated at the conclusion of the report.

A research project can also be just one phase of a larger project. After the reevaluation, a decision has to be made to continue the project or to make an adjustment in the design based on the previous results. If an adjustment in the design is made, then the second phase is treated separately because the design has been altered.

CONCLUSIONS

The intent of this chapter was to present research as clinical practice by comparing the research process to the occupational therapy process in the context of the problem-solving approach. It was suggested that developing a research project is just one step of a research continuum, beginning with the research consumer. The most important aspect of moving from "thinking" to "doing" is to develop a mind-set that assists the integration of the research process into regular clinical routine, and to garner resources to assist in the conduct of research. The survival of the discipline of occupational therapy depends upon the continuation, refinement, and expansion of the conceptual basis and quality of service delivery by clinical research that develops theory and demonstrates effectiveness.

ITEMS FOR STUDY AND DISCUSSION

- How can research be integrated as a clinical practice issue?
- How are an occupational therapy researcher and an occupational therapy clinician similar?
- What are the stages in the problem-solving approach, and how are they related to research?
- What are the steps in designing and conducting a clinically based research project?
- How is a treatment plan similar to a research plan?
- What is the research "mind set" or tradition?

REFERENCES

Conine, T. (1972). Dilemmas of research in occupational therapy. American Journal of Occupational Therapy, 26(2), 81-84.

Crocker, L. (1976). Validity of certification measures for occupational therapists. American Journal of Occupational Therapy, 30(4), 229-233.

Crocker, L. (1977). Linking research to practice: Suggestions for reading a research article. American Journal of Occupational Therapy, 31(1), 34-39.

Ethridge, D. and McSweeney, M. (1970a). Part I: Introduction. Research in occupational therapy. American Journal of Occupational Therapy, 24(7), 490-494.

Ethridge, D. and McSweeney, M. (1970b). Part II: The hypothesis Research in occupational therapy. American Journal of Occupational Therapy, 24(8), 551-555.

Ethridge, D. and McSweeney, M. (1971a). Part III: Research design. Research in occupational therapy. American Journal of Occupational Therapy, 25(1), 24-28.

Ethridge, D. and McSweeney, M. (1971b). Part IV: Data collection and analysis. Research in occupational therapy. American Journal of Occupational Therapy, 25(2), 90-97.

Ethridge, D. and McSweeney, M. (1971c). Part V: Data interpretation, results and conclusions. Research in occupational therapy. American Journal of Occupational Therapy, 25(3), 149-154.

Ethridge, D. and McSweeney, M. (1971d). Part VI: Research writing. Research in occupational therapy. American Journal of Occupational Therapy, 25(4), 210-214.

The Foundation. (1983). Research competencies for clinicians and educators. American Journal of Occupational Therapy, 37(1), 44-46.

Hasselkus, B. and Safrit, M. (1976). Measurement in occupational therapy, American Journal of Occupational Therapy, 30(7), 429-436.

Kerlinger, F. (1973). Foundations of Behavioral Research. New York: Holt, Rinehart and Winston, Inc.
Kielhofner, G. and Takata, N. (1980). A study of mentally retarded persons: Applied research in occupational therapy. American Journal Journal of Occupational Therapy, 34(4), 252-258.

King, L. (1978). Occupational therapy research in psychiatry: A perspective. American Journal of Occupational Therapy, 32(1), 15-18.

Madsen, P. and Conte, J. (1980). Single subject research in occupational therapy: A case illustration. American Journal of Occupational Therapy, 34(4), 263-267.

Mitcham, M. (1985). Integrating Research into Occupational Therapy. Rockville, MD: American Occupational Therapy Foundation.

Rogers, J. (1982). Guest editorial: Educating the inquisitive practitioner. Occupational Therapy Journal of Research, 2(1), 3-11.

Thatcher, V. and McQueen, A. (1967). The New Webster's Encyclopedic Dictionary of the English Language. Chicago: Consolidated Book.

Weiss, M. (1977). Cooperative research in occupational therapy. American Journal of Occupational Therapy, 31(1), 44-45.

Yerxa, E. and Gilfoyle, E. (1976). Research seminar. American Journal of Occupational Therapy, 30(8), 509-514.

Chapter 4

Current State of the Art in Occupational Therapy

Charlotte Brasic Royeen

CHAPTER OVERVIEW

Given an introduction to the process of research, this chapter presents an identification and explanation of the current research tradition in occupational therapy by discussing data analysis procedures as well as research designs employed in published occupational therapy research. Further, the state of the art of data analysis procedures in occupational therapy is contrasted to other disciplines. A synthesis of these findings is presented with summarization of the strengths and weaknesses in occupational therapy research pertaining to data analysis procedures and, in part, design. Finally, recommendations about statistical knowledge necessary for research competencies in occupational therapy are put forth.

KEY CONCEPTS

- *Occupational Therapy Journal of Research* is the primary research journal in occupational therapy.
- There has been an increase in research activity in occupational therapy.
- The bulk of the statistical procedures employed in the occupational therapy literature may be categorized as basic.

- Occupational therapy research tradition is in the stage of "emerging expertise."
- Nonparametric statistical procedures may be part of the developing research tradition in occupational therapy.
- Variable specification may be part of the developing research tradition in occupational therapy.

PRESENT STATUS OF RESEARCH

In an investigation by Royeen (1986a), articles published in the *American Journal of Occupational Therapy, Occupational Therapy Journal of Research, Occupational Therapy in Mental Health, Physical and Occupational Therapy in Geriatrics,* and *Physical and Occupational Therapy in Pediatrics* over a five-year period were indexed according to whether or not the article was statistically based. (The *Journal of Occupational Therapy in Health Care* was not indexed since, at the time of review, it was a practice-oriented, and not a research-oriented, journal.) These journals were chosen since they were the mainstream publications related to occupational therapy during the time period of interest (1980-1984). The study was conducted by Royeen (1986a) in order to investigate, in part, the research tradition in occupational therapy. The number of

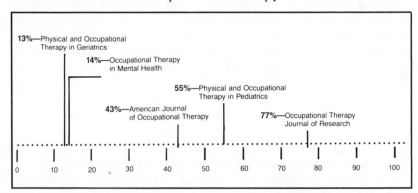

Figure 4-1. Continuum of research orientation of journals in Occupational Therapy (% of statistically oriented articles), 1980-1984.

60

statistically oriented articles within each journal was assumed to reflect the journal's research orientation and, therefore, a compilation of the indexing of statistical articles by journal was executed and is presented in Figure 4-1.

Considering Figure 4-1, it is apparent that *Occupational Therapy Journal of Research* is the most research-oriented journal in occupational therapy. This is consistent with the mission and purpose of *Occupational Therapy Journal of Research* as stated by West (1981) when the journal began: To provide a medium for the presentation and analysis of scientific activity in occupational therapy.

Journals dedicated to specialty areas of practice in mental health, geriatrics, and pediatrics follow a pattern speculated upon by clinicians: Pediatric practice, as reflected by *Physical and Occupational Therapy in Pediatrics*, is the most research based area of specialty occupational therapy. The argument that the joint occupational/physical therapy orientation of *Physical and Occupational Therapy in Pediatrics* skews its research orientation is moot since *Physical and Occupational Therapy in Geriatrics* is also a joint occupational/physical therapy publication, but it is not particularly research oriented.

Table 4-1 presents the overall figures for statistical vs. nonstatistical articles for all of the journals combined by years as reported by Royeen (1986a).

Table 4-1.
Frequencies Across Years (1980-1984), Totals and Precentage of Statistical Procedures for All Journals Combined

Category	Frequency by Year					Total
	1980 %	1981 %	1982 %	1983 %	1984 %	
Statistical Articles	33 (34)	35 (49)	47 (39)	52 (42)	51 (49)	218 (42)
Nonstatistical Articles	64 (66)	36 (51)	74 (61)	72 (58)	54 (51)	300 (58)
Totals	97 (100)	71 (100)	121 (100)	124 (100)	105 (100)	518 (100)

Table 4-1 reveals that, overall, there are more non-statistical articles than statistical articles in occupational therapy literature during this time period. One can surmise that since nonstatistical articles are the majority, research based articles are not the major influence in occupational therapy for this time period. Thus, in spite of the research orientation of leadership in occupational therapy, one can conclude that occupational therapy has yet to achieve a dominance of research in the journal literature.

Table 4-1 also reveals that from 1980 to 1984 for these five journals there has been an increase in the total number of statistical articles, with a corresponding decrease in nonstatistical articles. This finding is similar to that of Ottenbacher and Peterson (1985) who found an increase in the percentage of statistical articles in the *American Journal of Occupational Therapy* when all issues of 1983 were compared to those of 1973. Thus, it can be theorized that there is an increasing trend toward statistically based articles in the occupational therapy literature. It is assumed that the trend towards more statistically oriented articles reflects increased levels of research activity in occupational therapy. One may speculate that, even if there is not yet a dominance of research based articles in the occupational therapy literature, there has been a push toward a research tradition in occupational therapy.

Such conclusions are consistent with observations by individuals such as Acquaviva (1986) who note an increased research activity in occupational therapy. Increased levels of research activity in occupational therapy is noteworthy since the research orientation of the profession is fairly recent. However, a research orientation has been purpose-fully and deliberately fostered by the American Occupational Therapy Association as well as the American Occupational Therapy Foundation. The apparent increase in research activity suggests the the American Occupational Therapy Association and the American Occupational Therapy Foundation have successfully implemented strategies and procedures to promote research in occupational therapy. Thus, it can be concluded that (a) research activity has increased in occupational therapy and, (b) research is an emerging influence in occupational therapy.

DATA ANALYSIS PROCEDURES

In order to further evaluate and understand the current state of the art regarding research tradition in occupational therapy, statistically based articles were further reviewed by Royeen (1986a) to determine how often parametric or nonparametric data analysis procedures were used. A parametric statistical procedure can be defined as a statistical procedure that is based upon one or more assumptions about the underlying distribution or characteristic of the population from which estimates are obtained. Somewhat differently, "...a nonparametric statistical procedure ... has certain desirable properties that hold under relatively mild assumptions regarding the underlying population(s) from which the data are obtained" (p. 1, Hollander and Wolfe, 1973). Most importantly, "...nonparametric procedures forego the traditional assumption that the underlying populations are normal" (p. 1, Hollander and Wolfe, 1973). Considering that (a) little is known about the underlying distributions of variables of interest in occupational therapy (Royeen, 1986a) and (b) that researchers in occupational therapy and related fields conducting clinically based research admonish the predominate use of parametric procedures in lieu of nonparametric procedures (Bradley, 1978; Kirkpatrick, 1981; Lezak and Gray, 1984; Royeen and Seaver, 1986), it seems appropriate to assess differential use of parametric and nonparametric procedures in the occupational therapy literature.

Table 4-2.
Frequencies Across Years (1980-1984), Totals and Precentages of Parametric, Nonparametric and Nonspecified Procedures for All Journals

	1980 %	1981 %	1982 %	1983 %	1984 %	Total
Parametric Procedures	49 (91)	63 (79)	59 (76)	78 (81)	97 (84)	346 (82)
Nonparametric Procedures	4 (7)	13 (16)	15 (19)	17 (18)	12 (11)	61 (14)
Nonspecified Tests	1 (2)	4 (5)	4 (5)	1 (1)	6 (5)	16 (4)
Totals	54 (100)	80 (100)	78 (100)	96 (100)	115 (100)	423 (100)

Note: Nonspecified tests refer to correlations or tests of difference which were not specified by the author in the respective articles.
Note. Articles were indexed according to types of statistical procedures employed. Thus, one article could have more than one statistical procedures and accounts for a greater number of statistical procedures compared to the number of statistical articles.

Table 4-2 indicates that in the occupational therapy literature from 1980-1984 parametric procedures outnumbered nonparametric procedures at a ratio of approximately four to one. This finding may reflect the assumption among researchers that parametric procedures are "more powerful," and thus a "better" type of statistical procedure compared to nonparametric or robust statistical procedures. It may also reflect the research training that most research consumers and research therapists receive: A training which is oriented to parametric statistical procedures.

Given the prevalent use of parametric statistics, Table 4-3 presents the frequency and rank order of the particular parametric procedures found in the occupational therapy literature.

Table 4-3.
Summed Across Years (1980-1984)
and Rank Order of Parametric Statistical
Procedures for All Journals Combined

Procedures	Total Frequency	Rank Order
Pearson Correlation	74	1
Independent t-test	46	2
Factorial ANOVA	43	3
Chi Square	41	4
One Factor ANOVA	35	5
Post-hoc Multiple Comparisons	28	6
Paired t-test	24	7
Regression	14	8
Other	11	9
ANCOVA	10	10
Discriminant	5	11
Strudent t-test	4	12
Factor Analysis	4	12
Planned Contrasts	3	13
Meta Analysis	2	14
Canonical Correlation	1	15
MANOVA	1	15

Note: The "other" category includes infrequently indexed procedures such as path analysis, post hoc power analysis, multiple correlation analysis, Cronbach's Alpha and confidence intervals

COMPARISON TO OTHER DISCIPLINES

Table 4-3 shows that the ten most commonly employed parametric techniques in the occupational therapy literature are the Pearson Product Moment Correlation, the Chi Square*, the independent t-test, factorial ANOVA, one factor ANOVA, post-hoc multiple comparisons used with ANOVA, paired t-test, regression, analysis of covariance, and the category of other.

Based upon an adaptation of a classification scheme used by Goodwin and Goodwin (1985a), recategorization of the frequency of statistical procedures in occupational therapy literature into basic and advanced procedures is presented in Table 4-4. (The Pearson Product Moment Correlation, Chi Square, forms of the t-test, and the one way ANOVA were classified as basic techniques. Other procedures, such as regression and factorial ANOVA, were classified as advanced procedures.)

Table 4-4.
Basic Versus Advanced Techniques in
Occupational Therapy Literature

Category	Frequency	Percentage
Basic	224	67
Advanced	111	33
Total	335	100

Note: These calculations do not include the category of "other."

The Chi Square statistic is somewhat unusual in that it is commonly considered to be a nonparametric statistical procedure, yet it is often treated as if it were in a class of statistical procedure in and of itself (Feinstein, 1977). Furthermore, the Chi Square test statistic does have some distributional assumptions. For these reasons, it was categorized in parametric procedures, even though, strictly speaking, it is a nonparametric procedure.

Table 4-4 reveals that basic techniques are employed approximately 66% of the time, about twice as often as advanced techniques. Since the indexing methodology was essentially similar, comparisons can be made with the results presented by Goodwin and Goodwin (1985) when they indexed the literature of the American Educational Research Journal (AERJ) from 1979 to 1983. According to their definition, it was found that basic techniques comprised about 33% of the overall number of procedures used. Thus, occupational therapy research literature reflects the use of basic procedures more than literature in educational research at a ratio of approximately two to one. In all likelihood, a similar ratio exists in a comparison of field of occupational therapy to other disciplines such as medicine, psychology, and sociology.

In reviewing the educational psychology literature from 1979 to 1983, Goodwin and Goodwin (1985b) found factorial ANOVA, Pearson Product Moment Correlation Coefficient, and regression to be the three most frequently employed statistical procedures. When Edgington reviewed seven journals in psychology from 1948 through 1972, he found a marked increase in analysis using ANOVA, particularly factorial designed and repeated measures types. Thus, the analysis of research in educational psychology revealed more complex statistical procedures to be used, as compared to more basic procedures in occupational therapy. Again, a theme of emerging expertise in occupational therapy is evident. Table 4-5 presents a summary comparison of the most commonly used procedures in these two disciplines.

Table 4-5.
Comparison of Most Common Statistical Procedures
in Occupational Therapy and Educational Research

Rank Order	Occupational Therapy	Educational Psychology
1	Pearson Product Moment Correlation	Factorial ANOVA
2	Chi Square	Pearson Product Moment Correlation
3	Independent t-test	Regression

Furthermore, another review of Table 4-4 reveals that advanced procedures were employed in about 31% of the cases for all journals over this five year period in occupational therapy. Ottenbacher and Peterson (1985) similarly found that advanced procedures were used in 31.97% of the cases for articles in the American Journal of Occupational Therapy for the year 1983. Since the findings of these two separate investigations are similar, one may conclude that advanced statistical procedures account for a little less than one-third of the data analysis procedures employed in occupational therapy research.

The fact that the bulk of the data analysis procedures dealt with basic statistics, and that only one-third of the statistical procedures employed could be considered advanced, suggests that occupational therapy research is in an emergence period and not yet fully developed in terms of design, methodological, and statistical expertise. This impression is strengthened by a recent study by Johnson and Leising (1986). They conducted an analysis of citations in the *American Journal of Occupational Therapy* during 1978, 1980, and 1982 and found a "reliance on older literature" (p. 396, Johnson and Leising, 1986). The relative infrequency of recent citations suggests a lack of advanced level research development in the field of occupational therapy which is reflected in the methodology: The field does not yet have a strong and vigorous methodological tradition, but is in the stage of "emerging expertise."

To illustrate, many correlational investigations published in the occupational therapy literature which investigate test-retest reliability may be more appropriately investigated using research design and analysis procedures based upon analysis of variance (Cronback, 1947; Jackson and Messick, 1967). Similarly, many investigations employing multiple one factor ANOVA's can be more appropriately executed as factorial ANOVA's with subsequent multiple comparisons (Box, Hunter, and Hunter, 1978).

ANALYSIS OF NONPARAMETRIC PROCEDURES

Due to the previously cited importance of nonpara-metric statistical procedures in clinical research, the analysis of statistical procedures in occupational therapy was also extended into nonparametric statistics. Thus, frequencies of nonparametric statistical procedures were counted just as the parametric procedures had been counted. Table 4-6 presents the frequency and rank order of nonparametric statistical procedures in tabular form.

Table 4-6.
Frequencies and Rank Order of
Nonparametric Statistical Procedures for All
Journals Combined by Year 1980-1984

Procedures	Total Frequency	Rank Order
Mann Whitney U-Test	14	1
Spearman's Rho	11	2
Kendall Tau	8	3
Fisher's Exact Test	7	4
Kruskal-Wallis ANOVA	6	5
Wilcoxon Matched Pair Signed Rank Test	5	6
Split Middle Test of Trend	4	7
Cramer's V	3	8
Sign Test	1	9
Randomized Permutation Test (ANOVA)	1	9
Point Biserial	1	9

Review of Table 4-6 reveals that the five most commonly employed nonparametric procedures in the occupational therapy literature were the Mann Whitney U-test, Spearman's Rho, Kendall Tau, Kruskall Wallis ANOVA, and Fisher's Exact Test. The first four of these procedures deal with correlation and testing for differences between groups. Thus, the most commonly used nonparametric procedures are comparable to the most commonly used parametric procedures in occupational therapy literature, for those also dealt primarily with correlation and testing for differences between groups. Due to the similarity of function between the most commonly employed parametric and nonparametric procedures, one might surmise the bulk of the nonparametric procedures in occupational therapy literature could also be categorized as basic vs. advanced techniques.

In reviewing educational research literature, Goodwin and Goodwin (1985b) found the total percentage of nonparametric statistics to be ten percent. The percentage of nonparametric procedures reported by Royeen (1986a) is much higher at nearly 20%. Though each study reveals evidence of an increasing trend toward nonparametrics as identified by Borg (1984), the magnitude of the trend appears larger in occupational therapy research. The implication being that as occupational therapy builds a vigorous tradition of research methodology and continues to build a disciplinary data base, a significant component of it may consist of or result from nonparametric statistical procedures.

It must be noted that the process of developing a vigorous tradition of research in occupational therapy, i.e., of improving the quality and quantity of clinical research in occupational therapy, is complex. It will evolve uniquely, but will, in part, follow patterns and trends evidenced in other fields such as nursing (Bush, 1985). To illustrate, the controversy and discussion about methodologies as seen in educational research regarding quantitative vs. qualitative methodologies (Allender, 1986) may be mirrored in the development of a rigorous tradition of occupational therapy research.

However, a more central issue may evolve as identified by Litterest:

> The question is not one of qualitative or quantitative designs, it is one of commitment to disciplined inquiry and responsible clinical service (p. 604, Litterest, 1985).

Thus, the evolution of a strong methodology tradition in occupational therapy research will not be accomplished using a singular approach along one dimension, i.e., parametric vs. nonparametric procedures, qualitative vs. quantitative methodology, single case study research vs. group designs, and basic research vs. applied research. Rather, the development of a strong methodology tradition in occupational therapy will result from the synthesis or modification and refinement of a multidimensional approach to planning, executing, and analyzing research be it quantitative or qualitative.

For example, one preliminary step occupational therapy can take is the reconceptualization of the development of its data base (Gillette, 1982) to include variable specification. Variable specification within the data base of occupational therapy would consist of identification and compilation of the characteristics of variables of interest in occupational therapy using results from exploratory data analysis.

Exploratory data analysis refers to a set of procedures for screening research data prior to hypothesis testing. Occupational therapy clinicians are familiar with various types of screening tests for obtaining a quick estimate of whether some degree of abnormality or dysfunction is present in a particular client. However, occupational therapy researchers may be less familiar with an array of screening tests available for performing the same function on data sets acquired through research investigations: Data sets can be screened to explore their characteristics prior to inferential data analysis in the same way that the occupational functioning of clients is screened prior to full evaluation.

Screening tests for identifying the characteristics of data sets are known as procedures for exploratory data analysis (Hoaglin, Mosteller, and Tukey, 1981; Kotz and Johnson, 1982; McHill, Tukey, and Larson, 1978; Tukey, 1977), and these procedures were primarily developed by Tukey (1977). As the term implies, exploratory data analysis is a preliminary step conducted to determine what the data reveal: The process is designed to uncover the distributional characteristics of the data (Kirk, 1982). Procedures for exploratory data analysis are available in most statistical packages such as the Statistical Package for the Social Sciences (SPSSx) (Nie, Hull, Jenkins, Steinbrenner, and Bent, 1975) and the Statistical Analysis System (SAS) (SAS User's Guide, 1982).

Systematic and comprehensive collection of information from exploratory data analysis on variables of interest in occupational therapy would allow for thorough variable specification. Such a compilation over time would allow for a unique component of a data base within the field. It would enhance understanding of the variables of interest and have

71

implications for testing, measurement, and research in the discipline. It would also be the first systematic collection of such data within a discipline and may (a) accelerate the rate of research development within the field, and (b) set a standard for other disciplines to emulate.

THE EMERGING RESEARCH TRADITION IN OCCUPATIONAL THERAPY

In referring to research and educating researchers, Allender states, "Making decisions about methods is more difficult today than previously" (p. 174, Allender, 1986). Design and statistical procedures or methods are inexorably mixed; they each relate to the other and, it is the domain of methods and statistical procedures which will now be addressed.

Box (1984) discussed the general importance of practice in the development of statistical procedures. In occupational therapy clinical research, the relationship between practice, research design, and statistical procedures is crucial and underlies the future development of a tradition of research methods and practice unique to occupational therapy clinical research. The adequate development of such may be predicated upon fostering and generating research methods within the profession of occupational therapy, which in turn may be predicated upon an increased emphasis on graduate level education within the profession (Royeen, 1986b). It is impossible to facilitate the growth of a tradition of methodology on the part of research therapists in occupational therapy without support for graduate level education in methodology related to occupational therapy (master's and doctoral level). It is recognized that bachelor level training is simply not adequate for competency as a research therapist (AOTA, 1983), even though a research orientation for the research consumer can be fostered at the undergraduate level.

The following content is identified for competency of occupational therapists as consumers of research.

RESEARCH COMPETENCIES

Education, entry level and beyond, needs to include training in the following techniques so that practitioners can appropriately "consume" occupational therapy research, the majority of which will employ one or more of the following:

1. Pearson Product Moment Correlation;
2. Chi Square;
3. Independent, paired, and student t-test;
4. One factor ANOVA;
5. Factorial ANOVA with post hoc multiple comparisons;
6. Regression; and
7. ANCOVA.

Furthermore, in the primary professional journal for occupational therapists, *American Journal of Occupational Therapy,* approximately one of every five statistical techniques used is nonparametric. Thus, occupational therapy education, unlike many disciplines, requires a foundation in nonparametric statistics for consumers of research. Specifically, the following nonparametric techniques should be included in statistical training for entry level and continuing education:

1. Mann Whitney U-test;
2. Spearman Rho and Kendall Tau; and
3. Kruskall Wallis.

Additionally, the analysis of the state of the art of occupational therapy research has implications for the direction of the field. Since it appears that occupational therapy research is at a relatively basic level, it may be that the profession should now orient to, not just a research emphasis, but to an additional research emphasis committed to advancement of research past a basic level. More research in and of itself cannot move the field forward in the appropriate manner. Rather, more research at an advanced level is needed. This can most easily be accomplished via the following mechanisms.

1. Cultivation of promising occupational therapy researchers by continued and expanded financial support such as AOTF Doctoral Fellowships and AOTF research grants.

2. Promotion of research as a valid manifestation of the practice of occupational therapy. An example of this would be acceptance by fellow professionals as a "real ot" if one progresses directly through a bachelors, masters, and doctoral degree program without dropping out in order to practice occupational therapy clinically, i.e., acceptance of the research therapist.

3. Development of a research special interest section within AOTA so that those with common interests in research can develop support systems which are now currently available primarily outside of the profession.

4. Promotion of occupational therapy doctoral programs in conjunction with established and existing research programs in areas such as psychology, anthropology, educational research, and basic sciences.

5. Identification of respected and expert researchers in related disciplines who would be receptive to collaborative research and consequent followup by a promising or established occupational therapy researcher to initiate collaborative work.

6. Lobbying of local, state, and federal funding agencies for funding research in occupational therapy.

CONCLUSIONS

The field of occupational therapy is at a critical point regarding the emergence of a research tradition. It is an exciting and challenging time for all who are committed to the field. And, we can each play a significant role in the therapy. The specific role any of us will choose will depend upon individual interests, training and time. However, it is in the broad categorization of either research consumer or research therapist, or both, that we will continue the research tradition in occupational therapy.

ITEMS FOR STUDY AND DISCUSSION

Discuss the change in research orientation or research tradition in occupational therapy during the period 1980-1984.

- Why are nonparametric statistics important to occupational therapy?
- Discuss the differential use of basic and advanced statistical procedures in occupational therapy.
- Identify basic statistical competencies needed by the research consumer in occupational therapy.
- What is exploratory data analysis?
- How can variable specification further develop the discipline of occupational therapy?
- What are possible ways to further promote the research tradition in occupational therapy?

REFERENCES

Acquaviva, F.A. (1986). AOTA's Ad hoc Commission on occupational therapy manpower. American Journal of Occupational Therapy, 40(7), 455-457.

Allender, JS (1986). Educational research: A personal and social process. Review of Educational Research, 56(2), 173-193.

American Occupational Therapy Association (1983). Research competencies: For clinicians and educators. American Journal of Occupational Therapy, 37(1), 44-46.

Borg, W.R. (1984). Some important changes in educational research methods over the past twenty years. Paper presented at the Annual Meeting of the American Educational Research Association (New Orleans, LA, April 23-27).

Box, G.E.P., Hunter, W.G., and Hunter, W.G. (1978). Statistics for experimenters. New York: John Wiley and Sons.

Bradley, J.V. (1978). Robustness. British Journal of Mathematical and Statistical Psychology, 31, 144-152.

Bush, C.T. (1985). Nursing research. Reston, VA: Prentice Hall Co.

Comrey, A.L. (1985). A method for removing outliers to improve factor analysis results. Multivariate Behavioral Research, 20(3), 273-280.

Cronboch, L. (1947). Test reliability: It's meaning and determination. Psychometrika, 12, 1-16.

Edgington, E.S. (1974). A new tabulation of statistical procedures in APA journals. American Psychologist, 29, 25-26.

Feinstein, A. R. (1977). Clinical biostatistics. St Louis: C. V. Mosby Co.

Gillette, N. P. (1982). A data base for occupational therapy: Documentation through research. American Journal of Occupational Therapy, 36(8), 499-501.

Goodwin, L.D., and Goodwin, W.L. (1985a). Statistical techniques in AERJ articles 1979-1983: The preparation of graduate students to read the educational research literature. Educational Researcher, Feb., 5-11.

Goodwin, L.D., and Goodwin, W.L. (1986b) An analysis of statistical techniques used in the Journal of Educational Psychology 1979-1983. Educational Psychology, 20(1), 13-21.

Hoaglin, D.C., Mosteller, F., and Tukey, J.W. (1981). Understanding robust and exploratory data analysis. New York: Wiley and Sons.

Hollander, M., and Wolfe, D.A. (1973). Nonparametric statistical methods. New York: John Wiley and Sons.

Jackson, D.N., and Messick, S. (1967). Problems in human assessment. New York: McGraw Hill.

Johnson, K.S., and Leising, D.J. (1986). The literature of occupational therapy: A citation analysis study. American Journal of Occupational Therapy, 40(6), 390-396.

Kirk, R.E. (1982). Experimental design. (2nd ed.) Belmont, CA: Wadsworth Publishing Co.

Kirkpatrick, J.S. (1981). Nonparametric statistics: Useful tools for counselor. Personnel and Guidance Journal, 59(10), 619-651.

Lezak, M.D., and Gray, D.K. (1984). Sampling problems and nonparametric solutions in clinical neuropsychological research. Journal of Clinical Neuropsychology, 6(1), 101-109.

Litterest, T.A.E. (1986). A reappraisal of anthropological fieldwork methods and the concept of culture in occupational therapy research. American Journal of Occupational Therapy, 39(8), 602-604.

McGill, R., Tukey, J.W., and Larson, N.A. (1978). Encyclopedia of statistics. Boston, MA: Duxbury Press.

Nie, N.H., Hull, C.H., Jenkins, J.G., Steinbrenner, K., and Bent, D.H. (1975). Statistical package for the social sciences. New York: McGraw Hill.

Ottenbacher, K., and Peterson, P. (1985). Quantitative trends in occupational therapy research: Implications for practice and education. American Journal of Occupational Therapy, 39(4), 240-246.

Royeen, C.B. (1986a) An exploration of parametric versus nonparametric statistics in occupational therapy clinical research. Doctoral dissertation, Virginia Polytechnic Institute and State University, Blacksburg, Virginia. (University Microfilms International, Ann Arbor, MI: No. 8620659).

Royeen, C.B. (1986b). Entry level education in occupational therapy. American Journal of Occupational Therapy, 40(6), 425-427.

Royeen, C.B., and Seaver, W.F. (1986). Promise in nonparametrics. American Journal of Occupational Therapy, 40(3), 191-193.

SAS User's Guide: Statistics. (1982). Carey, NC: SAS Institute.

Sharrot, G.W. (1985). Ethics of clinical research. American Journal of Occupational Therapy, 39(6), 407-408.

Tukey, J.W. (1977) Exploratory data analysis. Reading, MA: Addison; Wesley Publishing.

Tupper, D.E., and Rosenblood, L.K. (1984). Methodological considerations in the use of attribute variables in neuropsychology/neuropsychological research. Journal of Clinical Neuropsychology, 6(4), 442-453.

Chapter 5

Future Trends in Occupational Therapy Research

Charlotte Brasic Royeen

CHAPTER OVERVIEW

The previous chapter presented an analysis of the current state of research in occupational therapy. A discussion of future trends and research traditions in the field is addressed in this chapter. In discussing future traditions, however, the chapter is limited to addressing trends regarding (a) the interpretation and the process of research, and (b) the politics and the impact of research. The potential future role of occupational therapy regarding these issues is identified and discussed.

KEY CONCEPTS

- Interpretation and research
- "Female" oriented thought processes
- Logic of justification - logical argumentation
- Politics and research
- Research utilization
- Research dissemination

OVERVIEW

According to Yerxa (1982), occupational therapy is politically threatened because our profession is at a vulnerable stage in developing and transmitting our body of knowledge. Developmental vulnerability is heightened during periods of transition, when one can forge ahead to higher levels of achievement or regress. During this transitional phase, our profession must forge ahead, with research as the vehicle through which professional development can reach new heights" (p. 594, Gilfoyle, 1986).

The development of research in occupational therapy during this transitional phase of the discipline as identified by Gilfoyle (1986) has been, in part, addressed by this book by delineating and promoting current research traditions. However, another critical issue concerning research has not yet been addressed: Future trends or traditions in occupational therapy research. Thus, this chapter will present an analysis of potential future trends based upon the previous analysis of current status of occupational therapy research as well as current status of related disciplines of academic thought. For example, what future trends are likely to influence occupational therapy research? What areas should the field of occupational therapy most critically and carefully address? Furthermore, if research is indeed the vehicle for professional development in occupational therapy as Gilfoyle (1986) proposes, how should the vehicle (the process of research) be modified, streamlined, or changed so that our developing body of research literature and research traditions do not become the "Edsel" of empirical investigation? Identification and consideration of these issues related to the future of research in occupational therapy could be the basis for another book. Thus, this chapter will be limited to the consideration of two primary areas regarding the future in occupational therapy research.

The two primary areas of future occupational therapy research which are to be addressed in this chapter may be categorized as (a) the interpretation and the process of research and (b) the politics and the impact of research. The former, the interpretation and the process of research, may be further broken down into categories of logical argumentation and cases. Similarly, the latter domain of politics may be further broken down into the categories of research utilization, dissemination, evaluation research, and public policy. Each of these domains and subcategories will be discussed in turn.

RESEARCH APPROACHES

There is an overall trend in academia toward positivism and holistic approaches in science (Winkler, 1985). These types of approaches can be assumed to be a future and important trend which will influence research in other fields as well as in occupational therapy. The current scholarly debate between qualitative vs. quantitative research methodologies (Smith and Heshusius, 1986) can be considered a product of the pressure brought to bear by the trend toward holism. However, the dichotomy of qualitative vs. quantitative research may be a luxury best left to academic theorists. For those who are more pragmatically oriented, the dichotomy need not be functional when one is most interested in the phenomenon to be investigated. Both sets of procedures, methodologies, and underlying conceptualizations are important and essential when one attempts to rigorously and validly study a phenomenon. Thus, the future trend in this area may be best served by attending to a research process germane to qualitative as well as quantitative research, yet neglected by each - interpretation. Interpretation transcends research methodologies. It concerns how one makes sense of or explains one's explanation of findings derived from either quantitative or qualitative research investigations.

To reiterate, interpretation is the process of understanding, explaining, relating, and integrating the findings of research. It is also the process of considering and explaining research findings in terms of context. For example, interpretation is the process of understanding a quantitatively oriented investigation beyond a pre-set "level of significance" or any other statistical standard. Furthermore, interpretation is the process of considering the findings of a qualitatively oriented research investigation beyond case replication, theme identification, or other qualitative method of data analysis. Interpretation is the process of checking if original assumptions underlying the research are valid. It is the process of relating facts, of identifying patterns, and of exploration to determine where findings can lead. Interpretation is a process which simultaneously produces a product - understanding.

Interpretation leads to understanding, which may be considered to be a product (comprehension or increased understanding of the phenomenon under study). It may be that emphasis upon interpretation as it pertains to all types of research, be it qualitative or quantitative, is the a trend and tradition for which occupational therapy researchers are best suited and in which occupational therapy researchers can set an exemplary standard. This may be so for a variety of reasons to be subsequently addressed.

Occupational therapy as a discipline is dominated by values, thought processes, and orientations associated with a "female" perspective. According to Scheuneman (1986), in methodology and statistics there are always problems with interpretations of outcomes, but a strength of the "female" thought process, such as the discipline of occupational therapy may have, is to view a problem in context. By viewing a problem or research results in context, i.e., related to its entirety or the part related to the whole, interpretation is correspondingly enhanced.

As a clinical practice profession, one of the strengths of occupational therapy has been an orientation to the whole person, i.e., of orienting to all domains related to a person's dysfunction (psychological, physical, and sociological). It may be that occupational therapy can generalize such a holistic orientation to research and employ a multifaceted orientation to the research interpretation process which could become part of the developing tradition of research methodology in occupational therapy.

The current emphasis on research procedures, research techniques, and research methodologies may be purposefully developed into an equal and innovative emphasis on interpretation of research findings: Perhaps the discipline can exemplify a paradigmatic shift in research which incorporates interpretation in a way that no discipline - even anthropology - has yet accomplished.

To illustrate, we have rules, history, and theory to guide us in the process of quantitative (Kirk, 1982) and qualitative (Kielhofner, 1982) research. Future research and tradition in occupational therapy might incorporate the development of rules, historical precedent, and theoretical rationale to guide the interpretation process of research findings to an extent beyond what is currently used and executed. Smith and Heshusius (1986) conjecture about this future trend and call it the logic of justification. They state the future orientation of research will "...focus not on techniques but on the elaboration of logical issues and, ultimately, on the justifications that inform practice" (p. 8, Smith and Heshusius, 1986).

Thus, future research tradition in occupational therapy may include, not just refinement and development of procedures appropriate for the execution of occupational therapy research, but also the development of a body of knowledge in yet to be developed and specified formats on how to interpret, i.e., the logic of justification or logical argumentation regarding the results and findings of research procedures (qualitative as well as quantitative) in occupational therapy research.

Logical argumentation as one category in interpretation is a process that will occur after the execution of occupational therapy research. Another subcategory of interpretation which, in and of itself, will constitute another methodology in future research trends is case analysis or a "cases-and-interpretation" process of research. Such a cases-and-interpretation methodology may be built upon the process of argument development used in the discipline of law (Caulley and Dowdy, 1986). A forerunner of the cases-and-interpretation model of research development has already been a mainstay in medicine evidenced by the work of such researchers as Rourke, Bakker, Fisk, and Stang (1983).

Yet, the process of cases-and-interpretation as a rigorous research methodology has not yet been fully developed and would allow for the modification and elaboration that occupational therapy could offer. To date, the work of Yin (1984, 1985, 1986) probably offers the most comprehensive delineation of aspects of the cases-and-interpretation methodology. Work in this area as related to occupational therapy research is in the beginning stages of development (Royeen and Fortune, 1987). The interpretation manual by A. J. Ayres (1976) is a developing example within the field of occupational therapy of a cases-and-interpretation model of research and serves as a forerunner for the development of this type of research in the field.

In the cases-and-interpretation methodology, and as seen in the Ayres manual (1976), each case is presented and interpreted. The collection of numerous cases constitutes what may be termed "a field of cases." Our future development - and one contribution to research methodology - may also lie in (a) developing guidelines for case selection; and (b) identifying and refining guidelines for how a field of cases, as a methodology, can be interpreted in the context of a clinic, school, or other grouping in society.

Another reason as to why the cases-and-interpretation methodology could be uniquely developed by occupational therapy has to do with the clinical orientation of the profession. The cases-and-interpretation methodology assumes a sample of cases purposefully selected. That is, cases are not selected at random but are selected according to some theoretical rationale. Such a sampling procedure does not force geographic spread and could allow for sampling within geographically restricted ranges. Thus, the cases-and-interpretation methodology could be built upon a clinical model: The clinical setting could provide the required subject sample. Such a research strategy would allow for proliferation of the clinician as a researcher paradigm by using a research design/methodology which fit clinical settings.

This discussion of the interpretation subcategories of logical argumentation and cases-and-interpretation deals with the conduct, product, or process of research. The next section of this chapter deals, not so much with the conduct of the research itself, but with the impact of the context of research surrounding any research endeavor, i.e., the political situation and the impact of research that must be addressed in a consideration of future trends.

There appears to be a "reductionistic" notion among occupational therapists that research, and research findings, represent an absolute truth. There is a belief that research findings are "pure" and represent a single reality devoid of political context. Thus, there has been an assumption underlying research development in our field that research is a non-political process.

The validity of this assumption is questionable. For there is always a political context to any research investigation, and to assume that it is not there is to assume research exists independent of context. To illustrate, one point of ethnographic research is to consider all of the realities surrounding the investigation of a phenomenon. It may be that future research in occupational therapy should always consider the political reality surrounding any and all occupational therapy research.

Therefore, one might express concern over the assumption that research will further develop the profession of occupational therapy and allow occupational therapy to compete for scarce dollars in the health care and education arena. This assumption is only partially true because it is necessary to consider and attend to the political context of all research, and as a future trend, the field of occupational therapy may choose to orient to the political context of research.

There are three subcategories to consider in the political context of occupational therapy research: research utilization, research dissemination, and modification of principles of evaluation research for use in occupational therapy.

According to Wilson (1985,) research utilization concerns how research findings are utilized or put into practice. Utilization of research appears to be a part of what Gilfoyle addressed in a recent article:

A major goal for this new era of creative partnership is the promotion of the profession through the integration of research and practice (p. 594, Gilfoyle, 1986).

Thus, research utilization is really orienting to how research results influence practice, which is - in fact - a political consideration. Political as used in this chapter refers to affairs of individuals, organizations, or governmental agencies. Research utilization has been defined by Ottenbacher, Barris, and Van Deusen (1986) as "...a complex process involving multiple components related to individual decision making, theory development, and the documentation of clinical practice" (p. 111).

Probably the best example of research utilization in occupational therapy is sensory integrative practice based upon the work of A. J. Ayres. One must wonder why.

How has her research made such an impact on practice?

What were the effective methods of communicating her research results?

How can research utilization in other areas of occupational therapy be equally as effective in practice?

By addressing these questions, successful dissemination mechanisms for occupational therapy research can be identified for study and modeling which may then effect future research in occupational therapy by supporting the research consumer. It is necessary to identify, modify, and strengthen research dissemination mechanisms in occupational therapy to further develop the tradition of the research consumer. Because research that is not used is rather like a piece of art which is not framed and hung for viewing, it may be well done, but it does not influence or effect people.

Consequently, our focus in research in occupational therapy must be linked with a concern for research utilization: Communication of the research findings for use by therapists (research consumers) must be a priority. However, research utilization is more than just communication of the research. It also includes the assurance of how the research results will impact the practice of occupational therapy and be used by practicing therapists.

The body of knowledge which pertains to research dissemination also pertains to research utilization. This is the second subcategory of the political context of occupational therapy. Yin (1986) states that applied research, unlike basic research, has as a primary goal the potential to influence practice or policymaking. Moreover, one must disseminate research findings in order to influence practice (the micro level) or policy (the macro level). Therefore, one must then consider, not just how the data or knowledge base will be developed in occupational therapy (Gillette, 1982), but also how that data base is going to be disseminated. Consequently, future traditions in occupational therapy research concern the diffusion mechanisms (Johnson, 1974), not just the research base. For, research can effect change in practice and policy only as far as it is influences practitioners and policymakers.

One type of research which considers dissemination on the same level and stage as design is evaluation research (Wholey, Scanon, Duffy, Fukemoto, and Vogt, 1971). Evaluation research, unlike experimental research, has a foundation of value judgments and political context. Modifying the aspects of evaluation research for use within the political context of occupational therapy research is the third subcategory to be considered.

It would not be appropriate for research in occupational therapy to adapt the value judgments inherent in evaluation research, but it may be prudent to modify and adopt some aspects of the of the political context inherent in evaluation research. Accepted guidelines for evaluation research are modified herein for infusion into occupational therapy research as an orientation to the political context of research. They are presented in Table 5-1.

Table 5-1.
Guidelines for Considering the Political
Context of Research in Occupational Therapy

Number	Guideline
1.	Who are stakeholders in the research (special interest groups, businesses, administrators, etc.) and why?
2.	Who are potential users of the research and why?
3.	What are ways to communicate with potential users of the research (stakeholders and policymakers) before, during and after execution of the research?
4.	How can community, organizational and professional support for the research be generated?
5.	What is the best medium for communication with those principle groups so identified?

The guidelines presented in Table 5-1 can be applied to occupational therapy research before, during, and after its execution. Also, the guidelines suggest that all research can be considered within the context of who will use it. Furthermore, consideration of the consumers of research will have an impact upon the conceptualization and implementation of the research as it is planned for dissemination. Thus, consideration of the political context of research is an inductive process with execution of the research.

The political act of planning research dissemination and specifically targeting policymakers is a valid and essential aspect of research development in occupational therapy (Royeen, 1986). More and more, direct consideration of policymakers is manifested in the occupational therapy literature, and it should be of increasing concern in occupational therapy research. To illustrate, Moersh stated:

> ... I suggest that occupational therapy re-
> search projects, such as the study of human occupa-
> tion planned by the AOTA Office of Professional
> Research Services, should include a stated intent to
> seek out and recognize implications of study findings
> or knowledge gained for public policy. Failure to use
> the knowledge gained from research in public policy
> would deprive members of society of their public
> good (p. 204, Moersh, 1986).

Such is the rational for a proposed tradition of political consideration in occupational therapy research: If one believes in the research, it is for the greater good that it be disseminated.

Influencing public policy requires a marketing approach as identified by Gilkeson (1985) and Hanft (1987).

Gilkeson identifies four steps in a systems approach to marketing which are herein adapted to apply for use with policymakers and presented in Table 5-2.

Table 5-2.
Guidelines for Research
Dissemination to Policy Makers

Number	Guideline
1.	State the research problem and plan.
2.	Determine policy personnel to be influenced.
3.	Evaluate past, present and future methods of communication effective with the identified policymakers(s).
4.	Plan a strategy of communication.
5.	Implement the strategy.
6.	Continually evaluate the effectiveness of the ongoing communication.

With such a strategy plan, one could attempt to accomplish with research what Masagatani (1986) terms "the expansion of occupational therapy markets."

SUMMARY

The coming years within the profession of occupational therapy will be a dynamic and changing period during which these projected trends may or not may become manifest. What remains to be seen is the role each of us will assume in developing the tradition of research in occupational therapy during this period of transition.

ITEMS FOR STUDY AND DISCUSSION

- Define and discuss interpretation related to research.
- How can a "female" perspective or thought process influence research interpretation?
- Define and discuss logical argumentation and cases-and-interpretation processes.
- Explain the relationship between politics and research.
- What is research utilization?
- What is research dissemination?

REFERENCES

Allender, J. S. (1986). Educational research: A personal and social process. Review of Educational Research, 56(2), 173-193.

Ayres, A. J., (1976). Interpreting the Southern California Sensory Integration Test Battery. Los Angeles: Western Psychological Services.

Caulley, D. N., and Dowdy, I. (1986). Legal education as a model for the education of evaluators. Educational Evaluation and Policy Analysis, 8(1), 63-75.

Dunn, W. (1985). Occupational therapy's challenge: Caregiving and research. American Journal of Occupational Therapy, 39(4), 259-264.

Gilfoyle, E. M. (1986). Professional directions: Management in action. American Journal of Occupational Therapy, 40(9), 593-596.

Gilkeson, G. E. (1985). Occupational therapy leadership potential can be developed through marketing techniques. Occupational Therapy in Health Care, 2(4), 91-94.

Gillette, N. P. (1982). A data base for occupational therapy: Documentation through research. American Journal of Occupational Therapy, 36(8), 499-501.

Hanft, B. E. (1987). The clinician as advocate for sensory integration. Occupational Therapy in Health Care, 4(2), 137-147.

Johnson, J. S. (1974). A descriptive analysis of the initial steps in the diffusion process for educational innovations utilizing state education agency personnel as linking agents. Unpublished dissertation, Open University, Washington, D.C.

Kielhofner, G. (1982). Qualitative research: Part one - paradigmatic grounds and issues of reliability and validity. Occupational Therapy Journal of Research, 2(1), 67-97.

Kirk, R. E. (1982). Experimental design: Procedures for the behavioral sciences. Belmont, CA: Wadsworth Press.

Masagatani, G. (1986). AOTA's ad hoc commission on occupational therapy manpower. Part 2: Summary of recommendations. American Journal of Occupational Therapy, 40(5), 525-527.

Moersh, M. S. (1986). Occupational therapy and public policy. American Journal of Occupational Therapy, 40(3), 202-205.

Ottenbacher, K. J., Barris, R., Van Deusen, J. (1986). Some issues related to research utilization in occupational therapy. American Journal of Occupational Therapy, 40(2), 111-116.

Rourke, B. P., Bakker, D. J., Fisk, J. L., and Strong, J. D. (1983). Child neuropsychology: An introduction to theory, research and clinical practice. New York: The Guilford Co.

Royeen, C. B. (1986). Evaluation of school based occupational therapy programs: Need, strategy and dissemination. American Journal of Occupational Therapy, 40(12), 811-813.

Royeen, C. B., and Fortune, J. C. (1987). Purposive sampling in clinical research. Paper presentation at the American Education Association Annual Meeting, April, Washington, D.C.

Scheuneman, J. D. (1986). The female perspective on methodology and statistics. Educational Researcher, June/July, 22-23.

Smith, J. K., and Heshusius, L. (1986). Closing down the conversation: The end of the quantitative-qualitative debate among educational inquirers. Educational Research, January, 4-12.

Wholey, J. S., Scanon, J. W., Duffy, H. G., Fukemoto, J. S., and Vogt, L. M. (1971). Federal evaluation policy: Analyzing the effects of public programs. Washington, D. C.: The Urban Institute.

Wilson, H. S. (1985). Research in nursing. Menlo Park, CA: Addison Wesley Publishing Co.

Winkler, K. J. (1985). Questioning the science in social science; scholars signal a "Turn to Interpretation." The Chronicle of Higher Education, June 26, 20-22.

Yerxa, E. J. (1982). A response to testing and measurement in occupational therapy: A review of current practice with special emphasis on the Southern California Sensory Integration Tests. American Journal of Occupational Therapy, 36(6), 399-404.

Yerxa, E. J., and Sharrot, G. (1986). Liberal arts: The foundation for occupational therapy education. American Journal of Occupational Therapy, 40(3), 153-159.

Yin, R. K. (1986). Knowledge Production and Utilization. Presentation for Research in the Education of the Handicapped Project Directors Meeting, Sponsored by the Division of Innovation and Development, U.S. Department of Education, July, 8, Washington, D.C.

Yin, R. K. (1985). Case Study Methodology. Presentation to the Institute for Special Education Studies, Sponsored by the Division of Innovation and Development, U. S. Department of Education, November 6, Washington, D.C.

Yin, R. K. (1984). Case study research: Design and methods. Beverly Hills: Sage Publications.

INDEX

impact of, 80, 86
importance of, 40-42, 85
increase in, 62-63
journals review, 60-62, 63-65
present status of, 60-63
reflective process in, 34-35
research competence, 73-74
research tradition development, 70-72,
73-74, 80, 82-84, 87
statistical procedures review, 63-68
training for, 64, 72-74
Occupational therapy theory research
investigation, 9-10
One factor ANOVA, 65, 66, 68, 73

Paired t-test, 65, 66, 73
Parametric data, 63, 64, 65, 66-68, 69
advanced procedures, 65-66, 68
analysis of covariance, 65, 66
ANCOVA, 73
basic procedures, 65-66, 68
Chi Square, 65, 66, 73
discipline comparisons, 67-68
in education research, 67
factorial ANOVA, 65, 66, 67, 68, 73
independent t-test, 64, 65, 66
journals review, 68
one factor ANOVA, 65, 66, 68, 73
paired t-test, 65, 66, 73
Pearson Product Moment Correlation
Coefficient, 65, 66, 67, 73
post-hoc multiple comparisons, 65, 66, 73
in psychology research, 67
regression, 65, 66, 67, 73
student t-test, 73
Pearson Product Moment Correlation
Coefficient, 65, 66, 67, 73
Peer review, 12-13
*Physical and Occupational Therapy in
Geriatrics,* 60, 61
*Physical and Occupational Therapy in
Pediatrics,* 60, 61
Positivism, 81
Post-hoc multiple comparisons, 65, 66, 73
Practice, 27-28
See also Clinical practice
Problem solving process, 42, 43, 44-45, 53,
55
occupational therapy process and, 42, 45,
55
research process and, 43, 45, 55
Psychology, 67
Purdue Pegboard Test research investigation,
9
Quality of life research investigation, 8-9
Quality research components, 7-14
absence of critical flaw, 12-13
clear communication, 13-14
common sense, 11-12

competence, 9-10
comprehensiveness, 9
context, 11
cost effectiveness, 10-11
creativity, 10
critical issue, 8-9

Regression, 65, 66, 67, 73
Research, 4
as absolute truth, 84
applied, 4-6, 7, 86
basic, 4-6, 7, 86
clinical, 6, 7
critical flaws in, 12-13
development of, 27-28
ethnographic, 84
evaluation, 80, 85, 86-87
experimental, 86
holistic viewpoint of, 82
humanistic orientation of, 27
impact of, 80, 86, 87-88
imperfect examples of, 13
importance of, 1-4, 14-15, 40
judgment decisions, 7-8
peer review of, 12-13
qualitative *vs.* quantitative, 81, 82
training in, 34
See also Humanistic research;
Occupational therapy research;
Problem solving process; Quality
research components
Research design, 7, 10, 46, 68, 72
author request letters, 48
in clinical setting, 84
collection of unpublished materials, 48
continuation of research project, 54
data analysis, 51, 53-54
data collection management, 50, 52, 53
data interpretation, 53-54
data synthesis, 54
delineation from, 48, 50-52
development of, 27-28
development of research questions, 49-50
documentation, 54
exploratory data analysis, 71
hypothesis, 50, 53, 54
implementation of, 53
instrumentation, 52
literature review, 47-49, 54
pilot project, 52
procedures description, 51
reevaluation, 53, 54
research issues identification, 49
resources identification, 49-50
second phase, 54
statistical procedures, 51, 53, 54
stroke design example, 52
subjects selection, 51
termination of research project, 54

93